The Emergency Medical Responder

Christian Ventura • Edward Denton
Emily Van Court

The Emergency Medical Responder

Training and Succeeding as an EMT/EMR

With Contributions by Pilar Nava-Parada

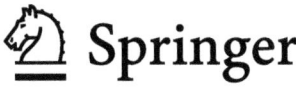 Springer

Christian Ventura
Boston University
Boston, MA
USA

Edward Denton
University of Arkansas at Little Rock
Little Rock, AR
USA

Emily Van Court
Simon's Rock EMS
Bard College at Simon's Rock
Great Barrington, MA
USA

ISBN 978-3-030-64395-9   ISBN 978-3-030-64396-6   (eBook)
https://doi.org/10.1007/978-3-030-64396-6

This Springer imprint is published by the registered company Springer Nature Switzerland AG
The registered company address is: Gewerbestrasse 11, 6330 Cham, Switzerland

Science Statement

This textbook conforms to the teachings, science, and recommendations of:

- National Standard Curriculum for EMT-Basic training by the National Highway Traffic Safety Administration (NHTSA)
- National Registry of EMTs Guidelines for Psychomotor Testing
- Emergency Cardiovascular Care CPR & First-Aid Guidelines by the American Heart Association and the International Liaison Committee on Resuscitation (ILCOR)
- Prehospital Trauma Life Support Guidelines by the NAEMT and the American College of Surgeons

This text may be suitable for use in the traditional EMT-Basic and EMR/CFR classroom with oversight of an authorized instructor. Appropriate medical direction, physician involvement, and consultation of local and state protocols are prerequisite to high-quality EMS training and supersedes the recommendations within this text. The guidelines, treatments, and methods in this text are in line with the most recent science by date of publication.

Editorial Science Support:
This text has been reviewed for scientific accuracy by Pilar Nava-Parada, MD, PhD. Dr. Nava-Parada is employed by Pfizer, Inc., and The Nava-Parada Family Fund Corporation

How to Use this Textbook

This textbook is intended to be used for:

- Complementing an EMT, EMR, or Certified First Responder course
- Studying for the NREMT exam
- Studying for a refresher for state licensure

This textbook is not particularly great for:

– Being used as a first aid manual
– Replacing emergency or medical services
– Use as a field guide in the middle of an emergency

In fact, you might want to call 911 again if you see your EMT flipping through the pages of this book before they treat you!

Acknowledgments

The authors wish to sincerely thank the following:
Christian Ventura

- Judith Inumerable, Ava Ventura, Xavier Ventura, Edith Inumerable, Steve Voorhees, family, and friends for continued support throughout the production of the book.
- Dr. Anne O'Dwyer, Dr. Francisca Oyogoa, Dr. Kathryn Boswell, Dr. Jessica Robbins, Dr. Diane Pirarino, Dr. Joseph Crouchman, Jesse Brady, and Caleb Sabatka for scientific and sociological support throughout my career, and embodying compassion, excellence, and kindness in everything.
- American Heart Association of New Jersey, Education Department at Hudson Regional Hospital, HAMES National, ACTSquad, and First Branch Ambulance for fostering kind support in my projects.
- My favorite partner Liz Connor, Christopher Knauth, Dr. Barnita Haldar, Dr. Charu Khatreja, Niviya George MPH, Saloni Jain MS, and my wonderful research assistants at the EMS lab.

Edward Denton

- Dr. Roy Denton, Eva Garcia CRNA, Reyes and George Hernandez, Reyna Rodriguez, Rebecca Rodriguez, and all family and friends for the moral support and encouragement all throughout life which has allowed for this current success.
- Alfonso Rodriguez and Raquel Rodriguez for providing the motivation to continue the pursuit of medicine and EMS education to save lives both directly through practice and indirectly through teaching.
- Sr. Angelina Pelliccia, Joan Tagliaferro, Dr. Jenna Winokur, Dr. Donn Winokur, Bryan Alban, Dr. Sarah Snyder, and Thomas Mulligan for creating and nurturing the seed, my interest and passion for science and medicine, that has led me to pursue it not only to the point I have reached now but even more into the future.

Emily Van Court

- Dr. Jesse Robbins and Dr. Katheryn Boswell for encouragement during hard times.
- Michelle Richards, Carl Vancourt, Eunseo Choi, and Roya Eshpari for being a supportive family throughout this process.

Additionally, the authors acknowledge that this work is that of the authors and does not reflect their institutional affiliations.

Introduction

Welcome to *The Emergency Medical Responder: Training and Succeeding as an EMT/EMR*! We are so glad to be joining you on your journey to becoming a healthcare provider. Allow us to be a few of the first people to welcome you to the best of both worlds—the healthcare professional AND first responder family. This book is gifted to you, the EMS student, to support you in becoming an evidence-based, compassionate, and patient-centered EMS provider.

What's So Unique About this Book

Unlike other EMS texts on the shelf, this book is special:

- It is the first of its kind to contain COVID-19 data and science from the pioneers of EMS pandemic response research.
- It follows a NEW outline for EMS teaching that makes concepts easy to understand, retainable, and applicable to the real world.
- The authors of this text are practicing EMS practitioners, instructors, and published scientists in emergency medicine.
- While remaining compliant with National EMS Curriculum Standards, this text acknowledges the latest evidence-based research on topics such as cardiocerebral resuscitation, double-sequentials, and longboard immobilization.
- This book is straight to the point, no mumbo jumbo, and no gimmicks.
- We address you intimately just as if you were one of our students in the classroom.
- We give you some of our tried and true tips for passing the Registry.

Contents

About the Authors

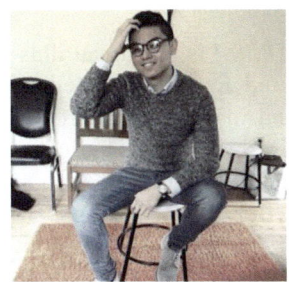

Christian Ventura, NREMT, EMS-I, RPhT, FHAMES is an EMS clinician, lecturer, and published researcher with an academic background in neuroscience and chemistry. He currently serves as the chairman of the Board of the Health Advocacy and Medical Exploration Society, Inc., on the Education Subcommittee of the Emergency Cardiovascular Care (ECC) Committee, and as the former advocacy chair of the American Heart Association ECC Committee Founders Affiliate. Christian has been involved in local, state, and national grassroots advocacy efforts for public health–related legislation and received the Heartsaver Hero Award in 2018. In 2020, Christian served as principal investigator for multiple studies investigating EMS pandemic response to COVID-19 in the United States. He is currently the State of Vermont advocacy coordinator for the National Association of EMTs. With his experience of teaching EMS providers from all backgrounds, he carries personal sentiment to this book to help grow the next generation of evidence-based and patient centered EMS providers.

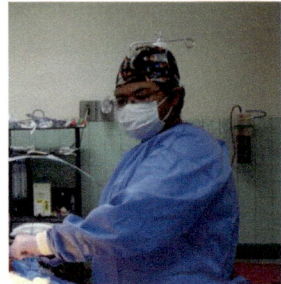

Edward Denton, NREMT, EMS-I is the director of education at the Health Advocacy and Medical Exploration Society and a certified instructor as well as instructor trainer through the American Red Cross, American Safety & Health Institute, and American Heart Association where he oversees continued compliance of CPR, first aid, and pre-hospital care programs. He also continues to work as an EMT in various agencies throughout the country. Whenever he can, Edward enjoys going to provide medical support on mission trips to children in countries such as Ecuador. His hobbies include international food tasting and creating ceramic art. He also enjoys visiting friends in Rhode Island.

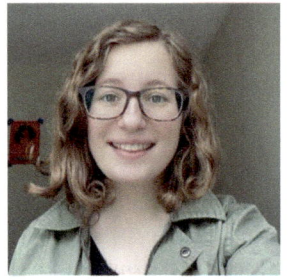

Emily Van Court, NREMT, EMS-I is a medical illustrator and Nationally Registered Emergency Medical Technician. With a background in cultural anthropology, she is also a lecturer in EMS and serves as deputy captain at her local EMS agency. She currently serves as the lead Institutional Review Board (IRB) correspondent and Qualitative Researcher at the EMS Pandemic Response Research Lab.

Chapter 1
The EMS System

Introduction

The US emergency medical services (EMS) system is a complex infrastructure of collaborative personnel that varies greatly by each state. Although fundamental principles are shared by EMS providers across the nation, methods of assessment, treatment, and transport often rely on posted local and state protocols. In this chapter, we will discuss the inner workings of the EMS system. By the end of this chapter, you will understand the scope of practice and role of a BLS provider, the chain of survival, and the critical role of medical direction.

Scope of Practice

Learning Objectives
Upon completing this section, you should be able to

- *understand* the BLS scope of practice,
- *identify* the different roles of EMS providers,
- *infer* your own role in the EMS system,
- *communicate* when advanced support may be needed.

In the US EMS system, we often differentiate EMS providers into two categories based upon their *scope of practice*, which outlines a healthcare provider's permitted actions, procedures, and process as prescribed by applicable law. As a soon-to-be EMS provider, you will obtain a scope of practice upon completing your course, passing several exams, and obtaining licensure by your state's department of health or equivalent. The *basic life support* (*BLS*) scope covers the assessment, treatment, and transport of sick or injured patients using noninvasive and nonsurgical techniques, although there are some exceptions to this (i.e., the use of an epinephrine auto-injector to treat a patient with acute anaphylaxis).

Examples of BLS providers include the following:

− Emergency medical responders (EMRs), certified first responders (CFRs), medical first responders (MFRs), or emergency trauma technicians (ETTs)
− Basic emergency medical technicians (EMT-Bs)

The *advanced life support* (*ALS*) scope involves the assessment, treatment, and transport of sick or injured patients using a combination of noninvasive and invasive procedures (i.e., starting an intravenous (IV) line in a patient's arm) with the help of advanced diagnostic tools (i.e., ECG monitors).

Examples of ALS providers include the following:

− Emergency medical technician intermediates (EMT-Is)
− Advanced emergency medical technicians (AEMTs)
− Paramedics (EMT-Ps)

Common EMR psychomotor skills

Airway

  − Use of oropharyngeal airway adjuncts
  − Suction of the upper airway

Breathing

  − Use of supplemental oxygen therapy
  − Use of positive pressure ventilation via bag valve mask ("BVM")

Circulation

  − Use of an automated external defibrillator
  − Use of prescribed auto-injectors
  − Hemorrhage control

Disability

  − Emergency lifting and moving
  − Cervical spine immobilization
  − Manual stabilization of suspected fractured extremities

Common EMT psychomotor skills

Airway

- Use of oropharyngeal and nasopharyngeal airway adjuncts
- Suction of the upper airway

Breathing

- Use of supplemental oxygen therapy
- Use of positive pressure ventilation via bag valve mask ("BVM")

Circulation

- Use of an automated external defibrillator
- Use of prescribed auto-injectors
- Administration of aspirin and oral glucose
- Hemorrhage control

Disability

- Emergency lifting and moving
- Cervical spine immobilization
- Manual stabilization of suspected fractured extremities
- Assist administration of prescribed medications

Paramedics are traditionally the highest ranking EMS provider and can perform advanced procedures such as performing endotracheal intubation, administering pharmacology intravenously, and analyzing cardiac rhythms.

Scope of practice can be expanded or limited by appropriate authorities, such as a state department of health. Regardless, BLS and ALS providers both require medical direction, often referred to as *medical control*, to carry out their scope of practice. Medical control is a method of physician involvement that assures high-quality care is provided to each and every patient.

There are two types of medical control:

- *Offline medical control* involves standing orders prescribed by the medical director of an EMS agency or receiving treatment facility.
- *Online medical control* involves real-time physician intervention where providers can request consultation and assistance in treatment/assessment over the radio or by phone.

Most 911 systems allow BLS providers the option to request ALS personnel if a patient's airway, breathing, and/or circulation is severely compromised. Dispatchers that respond to 911 calls operate at *public safety answering points (PSAPs)* and are able to dispatch police, fire, EMS, and other emergency services 24/7.

Check Your Understanding: *Medical Control*
You are currently assessing an 87-year-old patient that is currently taking a prescribed medication you have never heard of before. You are unsure whether this drug may pose as a contraindication. Which type of medical control should you initiate?

Medicolegal and Ethical Considerations

Learning Objectives
Upon completing this section, you should be able to

- *understand* legal and ethical considerations of EMS,
- *identify* levels of patient consent,
- *infer* the presence of unethical practices,
- *communicate* patient information confidentially.

State laws surrounding EMS duties and expectations are (in most cases) very similar throughout the United States. While on duty, EMS providers have a duty to (1) act, (2) perform a rapid yet thorough assessment in accordance with local protocols, (3) render appropriate care and treatment, and (4) transport sick or injured patients to a medical facility if necessary. The *duty to act* concept is a legal principle that mandates on-duty providers to render appropriate and expeditious care to a living patient so long as it is safe to do so. Off-duty providers are recognized as regular civilians and are only required to reasonably reduce harm of a patient and the general public. Noncompliance with the duty to act principle, deviations from standards of care, and any action that results in further illness or injury to a patient are all considered forms of *negligence*. Any action that causes injury or illness due to a breach of duty is known as *proximate cause*. *Abandonment* occurs when a provider terminates care without assuring appropriate continuity of care.

EMS providers also have ethical responsibilities while acting in official capacity and in some cases may be enforceable in accordance with applicable legislation. As an EMS provider, you have an ethical responsibility to

- be honest and transparent in all forms of communication, documentation, and reporting;
- keep up to date by pursuing continuing education opportunities and mastering all BLS skills;

– conduct regular debriefs and self-assessment and pursue methods to reasonable improve one's performance and positively affect patient outcomes;
– prioritize the emotional, physical, and mental needs and concerns of patients.

In order for a provider to initiate assessment and care of a patient, *consent* must be properly obtained, which is legal permission on behalf of the individual to receive emergency medical services.

EMS providers can obtain consent in two ways:

– *Expressed consent* is obtained when a conscious competent legal adult with full decision-making capability agrees to receive the provider's services. The patient is required to be informed of the steps, risks, and benefits of each procedure.
– *Implied consent* is automatically obtained in the event that a patient is unconscious or has an altered mental status and operates under the assumption that the patient would consent to immediate emergency care.

If a conscious adult withdraws or does not give expressed consent to the provider, this is known as *refusal of care* and should be documented and recorded in accordance with your agency's protocols. Refusal of care may be obtained by the completion of an against medical advice (AMA) form, acknowledging the potential health risks of refusing EMS care. A patient has the right to refuse or withdraw consent at any given time. *Assault* occurs when a threat or attempted physically offensive action is made. *Battery* occurs when a patient is touched, treated, or assessed against their will.

Special considerations for obtaining consent:

– Consent from children must be provided by their parent or legal guardian **except** in the event that the child requires immediate emergency care. In this case, implied consent can be assumed. Refer to your local or state protocols regarding minors.
– Consent from adults without full decision-making capability must be obtained by their caregiver or other legal representing authority **except** in the event that the patient requires immediate emergency care. In this case, implied consent can be assumed.

Refusal of care considerations:

– Do your best to encourage the patient to seek emergency care, and thoroughly inform them of the potential risks of refusing care. You may have to ask more than once.
– Consult medical control or law enforcement if assistance is needed.
– Assure the patient has full mental and legal decision-making capacity.
– Obtain proper documentation of refusal of care.

When a patient, caregiver, or family member presents an official document that concisely conveys the treatments they would like to receive and which they would like to refuse in the event they cannot communicate their consent, this is known as an *advance directive*. Examples of advance directives include "Do Not Resuscitate" (DNR) orders and power of attorney. An advance directive generally requires a signature from the patient's physician and/or attorney. In the event a DNR is not appropriately presented in a timely manner, it is considered acceptable to attempt resuscitation efforts. Consult your local protocols for further guidance on DNRs and "Do Not Attempt Resuscitation" (DNAR).

EMS providers are legally obligated to protect and maintain *patient confidentiality*, which includes findings from any assessment, treatments provided, and medical history. Patient confidentiality is regulated in the United States by the *Health Insurance Portability and Accountability Act of 1996* (*HIPAA*). HIPAA assures that providers safeguard *protected health information* (*PHI*) that could be used to identify a patient. This type of information is called *personally identifiable information* (*PII*) and includes names, dates of birth, and social security numbers, among other categories. HIPAA violations are often accompanied by large fines, loss of employment, and in some cases imprisonment. The disclosure of confidential information to any party other than the patient or their legal caregiver must be facilitated by the use of an official release form. Release is not required, however, when health information is needed to be transmitted for the purpose of continuing care or in court testimony via a subpoena. Special circumstances where release of information may be necessary are called *special reporting situations*. Examples of special reporting situations include when a crime has occurred, such as sexual assault or domestic abuse.

> **Check Your Understanding:** *Medicolegal and Ethical Considerations*
> You are responding to the scene of a 15-year-old unconscious male who is not breathing. Are you permitted to render care? If not, why? If so, what type of consent might this be?

Chapter Summary

Section "Scope of Practice"
- The *basic life support* (*BLS*) scope involves a combination of the assessment, treatment, and transport of sick or injured patients using noninvasive and nonsurgical techniques, while *advanced life support* (*ALS*) includes additional invasive procedures such as IV access and endotracheal intubation.
- *Medical control* is a method of physician involvement that assures high-quality care is provided to each and every patient.

Section "Medicolegal and Ethical Considerations"
- In order for a provider to initiate assessment and care of a patient, *consent* must be properly obtained, which is legal permission on behalf of the individual to receive emergency medical services.
- EMS providers are legally obligated to protect and maintain *patient confidentiality*, which is regulated in the United States by the *Health Insurance Portability and Accountability Act of 1996 (HIPAA)*.

Tricks of the Trade
- Either it's in your written narrative or it didn't happen! You should prepare every patient care report as if you were to present it before a judge, because one day you might have to!
- When in doubt, contact medical control! There is no harm in asking for a consultation from a physician. In fact, you are encouraged to.

Practice Questions
1. What is adequate proof that a patient has a valid Do Not Resuscitate order?

    (a) You are presented with a DNR that has no provider signature.
    (b) The family of the patient on scene informs you that the patient has a DNR but it is unable to be presented at that time.
    (c) You are presented with a DNR, checked to confirm both the provider's signature and the signature of the patient.
    (d) The patient has a bracelet, not listed in local protocols, representing the DNR, letting you know that a patient has one.

2. You arrive on scene to a 35-year-old patient who is conscious and responding to questions. They appear to have a broken arm but are adamantly refusing treatment or any kind of assessment. Despite this, your partner begins to splint the arm. What legal consideration has your partner transgressed?

    (a) Battery
    (b) HIPAA
    (c) Assault
    (d) Neglect

3. Under HIPAA regulations, what information about a case is **not** protected?

    (a) The type of injury sustained.
    (b) The patient's name.
    (c) The patient's social security number.
    (d) The patient's physical description.

Chapter 2
Anatomy and Physiology for the Emergency Provider

Introduction

A basic understanding of the human body is crucial for any medical provider. As you encounter different medical emergencies, understanding the basic mechanics behind the affected systems and understanding how to effectively communicate the details of the emergency to other providers are essential in the field. This chapter will work toward the goal of communication as it covers the standardized terms for different ways to view the body, the standardized terms for describing placement in and on the body, and describing the body's position. This chapter will also work toward helping you understand the mechanics of the body as it covers major skeletal structures, cell biology, and how the body develops with time.

Planes and Perspectives

Learning Objectives
Upon completing this section, you should be able to

- *understand* how anatomical planes separate the body,
- *identify* the direction and placement of each anatomical plane,
- *infer* why planes are useful when viewing the body,
- *communicate* internal structures in relation to the anatomical planes.

Anatomical planes are different ways to divide and view the body. You can imagine each plane as cutting the body in half on different axes. You can use your understanding of these planes to help visualize the placement of internal structures in relation to these planes and each other.

Coronal

The coronal plane, or the frontal plane, runs through the body, dividing it into a front and a back half. So, once divided, the face would be separated from the back of the head.

Sagittal

The sagittal plane, or the median plane, runs through the body and divides the body into left and right halves. The left arm is on the opposite side of the plane as the right. This plane is perpendicular to the coronal plane.

Transverse

The transverse plane, or the horizontal plane, runs through the body horizontally, dividing the body into top and bottom halves.

Directional Terms

Learning Objectives
Upon completing this section, you should be able to

- *understand* how and why directional terms are used,
- *identify* the meaning of each directional term,
- *infer* the importance of standardized language in EMS,
- *communicate* positions on the body using directional terms.

Have you ever heard horror stories of doctors amputating the wrong leg or operating on the wrong organ? As an EMS provider, you won't be performing surgery or amputating any limbs, but being able to communicate a specific location on the body is still important. It is necessary for communicating both in the field and with any receiving medical personnel to ensure a seamless and efficient transfer. Position on the body is communicated using *directional terms*, which come in pairs and usually refer to one plane of the body.

Right and Left

Right and left are common terms that we use in everyday life and reference the two sides of the body. In medicine, right and left refer to the patient's right and left, not the provider's right and left.

Medial and Lateral

Imagine a line running straight through the middle of the body, from the top of the head to the navel. That line is the midline of the body. A part of the body that is medial is close to the midline of the body. Lateral is the opposite, meaning that a part of the body is an outer structure or far from the midline. These terms are used to define relations between different areas of the body. For example, the chest is medial to the arms (closer to the midline than the arms), while the arms are lateral to the chest (further from the midline than the chest).

Ventral and Dorsal

If someone is facing you, you are looking at the front of the body. Something toward the front of the body is considered ventral, also called anterior. Something toward the back of the body is dorsal or posterior. For example, on the foot, the toes are ventral and the heel is dorsal/posterior.

Superior and Inferior

A part of the body that is superior is closer to the head or higher in the body than what it is being related to. Inferior means that something is closer to the feet or lower in the body. For example, the mouth is inferior to the nose and the nose is superior to the jaw.

Proximal and Distal

These two terms are mostly used for structures on extremities. Proximal refers to a part of an extremity that is closest to the point where the extremity attaches to the rest of the body. Distal refers to a part of an extremity that is closest to the end of that extremity. For example, the hand is distal to the elbow and the shoulder is proximal to the elbow.

Superficial and Deep

You will hear these terms often when talking about the depth of cuts and lacerations. Superficial means close to the surface of the body, or the skin. Deep means further away from the surface of the body. For example, a scraped knee will be described as superficial, because the depth of the injury does not go much further than the surface of the skin, but a stab wound will be referred to as deep because the depth of the injury is much more extensive.

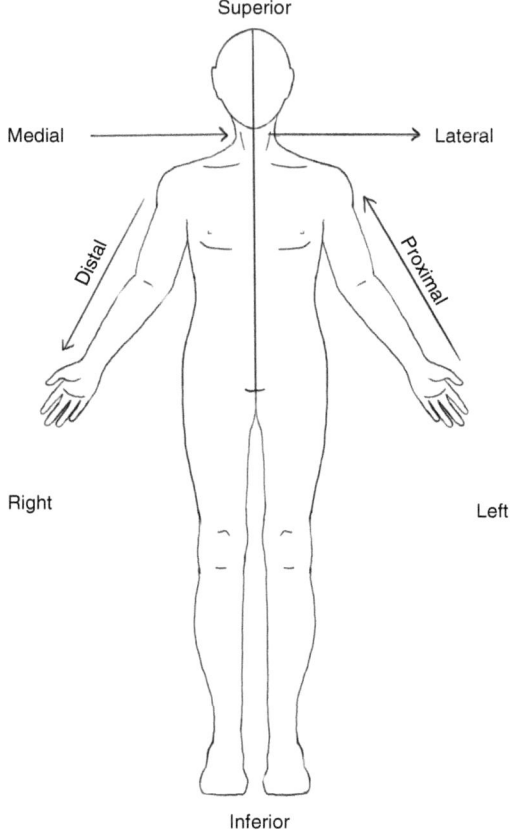

Positions

> **Learning Objectives**
> Upon completing this section, you should be able to
>
> - *understand* how each term relates to an anatomical position,
> - *identify* the anatomical position from viewing a patient,
> - *infer* different contexts in which each position will be present,
> - *communicate* a patient's position with the correct term.

Anatomical positions refer to the position a body is in and are important to document, as these positions can give providers a lot of clues to the state of their patients. For example, if a patient is sitting up when you get to a scene, you can rule out some mechanisms of injury: it is unlikely that they fell or had a high force impact. So, even if the patient cannot communicate, the position itself gives clues to what type of emergency a patient is having and how you should proceed with care.

Supine
The supine position refers to a person who is lying on their back, facing upward. So, if you come on scene to a patient lying on their back on the floor, you would document them as being supine.

Prone
The prone position is the opposite of supine. It refers to a person lying facedown, with their back facing upward.

Fowler
Fowler's position is when patients are sitting up at or close to a 90-degree angle. So, if you walk on scene to a patient sitting up in a chair, they would be in Fowler's position.

Semi-Fowler
Semi-Fowler's position refers to when a person is sitting with their back raised at a 45-degree angle. Most commonly, the back of stretchers will be set to 45 degrees when transporting patients to achieve this position and help the patient with breathing and comfort during transport.

Trendelenburg
The Trendelenburg position is the opposite of semi-Fowler's position. Instead of the head and back being elevated, the feet are elevated at or close to a 45-degree angle. So, a person lying on the floor while propping their feet on a chair is considered to be in the Trendelenburg position.

Lateral Recumbent
The lateral recumbent position refers to a person who is lying on their side. Depending on which side they are lying on, they could be in the left or the right lateral recumbent positions. The left lateral recumbent position is also known as the recovery position or a position utilized to open the airway. More details on the recovery position will be discussed in later chapters.

Major Skeletal Structures

Learning Objectives
Upon completing this section, you should be able to

- *understand* the purpose of the skeletal system as a whole,
- *identify* the different major skeletal structures,
- *infer* the purpose of each bone within the skeletal system,
- *communicate* the proper name and placement of different skeletal structures.

The *skeletal system*, made up of bones and joints, serves many functions in the body. First and foremost, it serves as the body's frame, providing structure and stability. Muscles attach to and form around this frame to allow for movement at the joints. The bones themselves have a few additional functions, such as producing red blood cells. In total, an adult skeleton has 206 bones divided into the axial and appendicular skeletons. However, for the purposes of emergency response, you will only have to memorize about a dozen.

Axial Skeleton

The axial skeleton can be thought of as the "trunk" of the body, as it encompasses the head and torso. More specifically, the axial skeleton refers to the skull, the bones around the thoracic cavity, and the spinal cord.

Skull

The *skull* protects the brain and the upper airway. The bones that make up the skull can be split into two categories, the *cranial bones*, referred to collectively as the cranium, and the *facial bones*. The cranium is made up of plates fused together to form the top of the skull.

Cranial Bones

The *frontal bone* is the plate that makes up the forehead.

The *parietal bones* make up the very top of the skull, and there are two, one on the left and one on the right.

The *temporal bones* lie behind the ears and make up the lower side of the skull. Like the parietal bones, there is one on each side of the skull.

The *occipital bone* makes up the base of the skull.

Facial Bones

The *maxilla* is the upper jaw. The bones that make up the maxilla are fused to the rest of the skull.

The *mandible* is the lower jaw which, unlike the fixed maxilla, is attached to joints that allow it to move.

The *zygomatic bones* are more commonly referred to as the cheek bones and lie above the upper jaw.

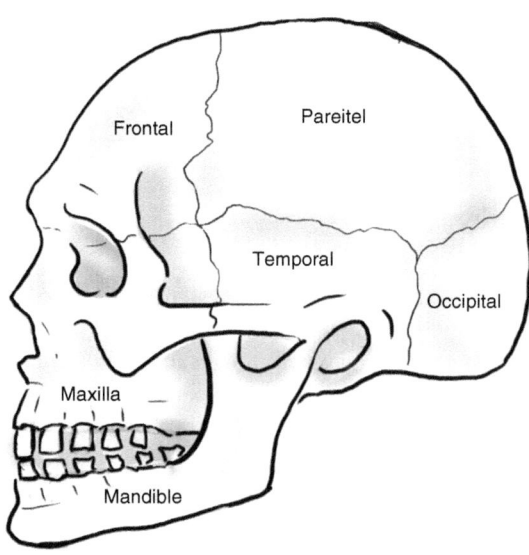

Thoracic Cage

The thoracic cage, more commonly known as the rib cage, makes up the chest. Its main purpose is to protect the essential organs that lie in the thoracic cavity, such as the heart and lungs.

The *ribs* make up the body of the rib cage. There are 12 pairs of ribs, 10 of which are connected to the sternum with cartilage and the lowest 2 which are free-floating.

The *sternum*, commonly known as the chest bone, is a plate that lies in the middle of the chest and helps protect the heart and stabilize the ribs.

The *xiphoid process* is a small bone connected to the end of the sternum. It has no known function but is important to know because of the dangers associated with it. It can be disconnected from the sternum due to trauma and puncture the organs in the thoracic cavity.

Spinal Column

The spinal column, or the backbone, is the main support for the body and houses the pathway for the nerves to branch out from the brain to the rest of the body. The bones that make it up are called vertebrae. The importance of the spinal column makes it one of the top priorities when caring for patients, as damage can result in paralysis or death. The higher up in the column the damage is, the more the body is at risk for paralysis through those nerve pathways being cut. The spine is split into five sections.

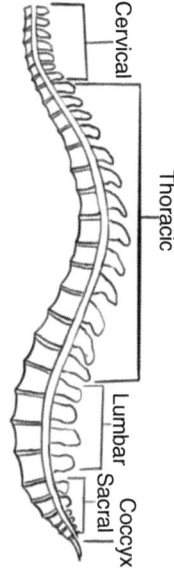

The *cervical spine* is the section of the spine that makes up the neck. It is made of seven vertebrae.

The *thoracic spine* makes up the upper back and is made of 12 vertebrae.

The *lumbar spine* makes up the lower back and is made of five vertebrae.

The *sacrum* extends into the pelvis and is made of five fused vertebrae.

The *coccyx*, known as the tailbone, is made of four fused vertebrae.

Appendicular Skeleton

The appendicular skeleton makes up the extremities and the joints which attach them to the trunk of the body. The joints provided by the appendicular skeleton allow for most motion to occur, such as walking and any movement of the arms. A good way to categorize the bones that make up the appendicular skeleton is into bones associated with the upper extremities and those associated with the lower extremities.

Upper Extremities

The upper extremities include both arms and the shoulders. The shoulders hold the joint which attaches the arms to the trunk of the body.

The *scapula*, also known as the shoulder blade, connects with the clavicle to form the shoulder girdle, connecting the arm to the rest of the body.

The *clavicle*, also known as the collarbone, is a long bone that forms another part of the shoulder girdle. It is a bone that is easily broken, so it is important to remember once you learn how to stabilize breaks.

The *humerus* is the long bone that forms the upper arm.

The *radius* is one of the two long bones in the lower arm. It runs along the same side of the arm as the thumb.

The *ulna* is the other long bone in the lower arm that runs opposite to the radius.

Lower Extremities

The bones in the lower extremities include the pelvis, legs, and feet.

The *pelvic girdle* holds three different pairs of bones, the pubis, ischium, and ilium. You don't need to remember these, but it is important to know that they fuse to create the pelvis.

The *femur* is the long bone that forms the thigh. It is one of the thickest bones in the body and very difficult to break. This is because it provides stability and protects the femoral artery.

The *patella* makes up the kneecap and is one of the bones that can be dislocated.

The *tibia* is the forward-most bone in the lower leg.

The *fibula* is the other long bone in the lower leg.

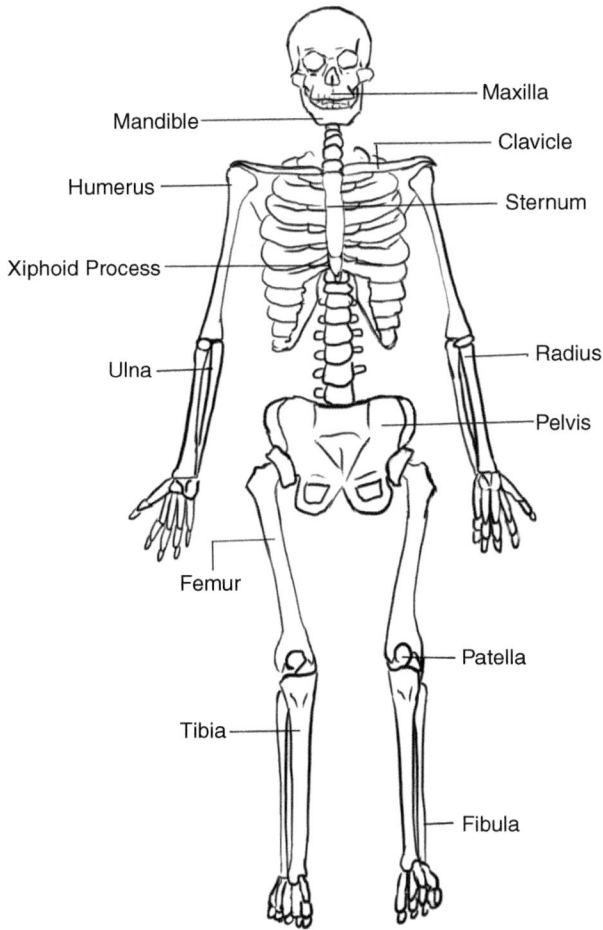

Human Development

Learning Objectives
Upon completing this section, you should be able to

- *understand* how the body changes as a person ages,
- *identify* the major stages in life,
- *infer* the connections between physical and psychological changes,
- *communicate* appropriately for each age group.

As humans age, our bodies and minds develop and change. These physiological changes greatly affect human anatomy and, therefore, how each age group responds to emergency situations, both physically and mentally. As EMS providers who have to assess and treat patients of all ages, it is important to know these changes and the characteristics of people in different age groups. This understanding allows providers to cater their care to their specific patient's needs. There are eight main age groups, based off of Erikson's stages of development, with distinctive characteristics that are important to be able to distinguish.

Infants (0–1 Years)
This category includes the subcategory of *neonates*, which encompass infants in their first month of life.

Physically, normal vitals within this age range fluctuate greatly. The pulse slows from 90–180 BPM at birth to 100–160 BPM throughout the first year. Neonates have a normal respiration rate of 30–60 RPM that slows to 25–50 RPM throughout the rest of infancy. From the first month of life onward, the older the patient is, the lower the heart rate and respiration rate are expected to be. The opposite is true for blood pressure; neonates are expected to have a systolic pressure of between 50 and 70 mmHg, and that increases to 70–95 mmHg within the rest of the first year.

Other physical characteristics of this age group can be found within the respiratory and skeletal systems. During infancy, respiratory issues are much more common than they are later in life. This is partly because infants' heads are very large in proportion to their bodies and lower airway, so it is very easy for their head to be wrongly positioned, causing an airway obstruction. Tongues are proportionally larger in infants and can also cause an airway obstruction. Upper airway aside, infants' lungs are also more delicate than those of adults, so overventilation on the part of the EMS provider can be dangerous. Skeletally, the bones in the skull have not yet fused in early infancy, causing two soft spots, called *fontanelles*, on the top and back of the head that providers should be cautious of. Sunken fontanelles can be a good indicator of dehydration in infants.

Psychologically, infants are just starting to experience and interact with the world around them. Communication is nonverbal, but rather, emotions are expressed through behaviors such as crying. Later in infancy, different forms of attachment with caregivers start to settle. This may translate into emotions like separation anxiety or distress at distance put between the infant and their caregiver, which you, as an EMS provider, will need to work around.

Toddlers (1–3 Years)
Physically, heart rate has lowered compared to infancy, normally being 90–150 BPM. The normal respiration rate has also slowed to 20–30 RPM, and their respiratory systems have become more developed as a whole, although the head to body proportion poses a similar problem as it did in infancy. Following the previously established trend, the systolic blood pressure in this age group increases to 80–100 mmHg. Something to note as well is that toddlers have developing immune systems and have lost the passive immunity gained in utero. Therefore, they are very susceptible to viruses.

Psychologically, this is the age where separation anxiety peaks. As an EMS provider of a patient this age, prepare to have to interact with the caretakers of the toddler and have to communicate with them throughout responding to the emergency. At this age, toddlers are beginning to develop language, but cannot yet utilize full sentences or abstract concepts.

Preschoolers (3–6 Years)
Physically, the normal heart rate has lowered compared to toddlers, to around 80–140 BPM. The normal respiration rate has also slowed to 20–25 RPM. The head to body proportion is still exaggerated compared to adults. Continuing the trend, the systolic blood pressure in this age group increases to 80–100 mmHg.

Psychologically, preschoolers are beginning to learn more about interpersonal connections and at this age can communicate using full sentences. Explaining to and interacting with patients this age and above are important. You should not direct all attention to the caretakers.

School Age (6–12)
Physically, the normal range of heart rate slows to 70–120 BPM, and the respiration rate slows to 15–20 RPM. Systolic blood pressure increases to 90–110 mmHg. The head to body proportions that affected the respiratory system previously also start to normalize into adult proportions.

Psychologically, this is the period where children start to develop self-esteem and more complex forms of reasoning. You should interact directly with these patients and keep in mind their developing self-esteem during those interactions.

Adolescents (12–18)
Physically, adolescents are stabilizing into their adult bodies. Vitals and mental states are leveling off. Heart rate is normally 60–100 BPM, and respiratory rate is 12–20 RPM, both of which you may notice are the adult range. Systolic blood pressure is normally between 90 and 110 mmHg. Adolescents experience a lot of growth, and the reproductive system develops to maturity.

Psychologically, adolescents begin to strive for independence and self-expression. As adolescents begin searching for identity, there is a risk of depression and suicidal thought. During this time, it is important to respect the patient's modesty and keep their mental health in mind. While this is always true, it is especially important in this age group and older.

Young Adults (19–40)
Physically, the body and vital signs stop fluctuating and normalize. Heart rate is 60–100 BPM, respiration rate is 12–20 RPM, and systolic blood pressure is 90–140. Toward the end of this period, symptoms of aging start to occur, such as slow reflexes and less muscle density. Lifestyle and habits, such as eating, exercising, and drug use, start to affect the health of the patient.

Psychologically, the mental state starts to level out as well. Stress is a large factor of the adult brain as adults start to juggle different aspects of life, such as work and family.

Middle Adults (41–60)

Physically, vitals are the same as those of young adults. The main physical difference is that the risk of cardiovascular issues begins to peak. During this time period, menopause and infertility may begin to affect female patients. Also, this age group is at risk for a decline in hearing and sight.

Psychologically, this age group tends to be the most stable aside from stress from financial and family issues.

Older Adults (61+)

Older adults have begun to decline physically, and vital signs are difficult to average due to the variety of illnesses that affect this population. The baseline vitals used for assessment should be the same as those used for earlier stages of adulthood. Each body system starts to decline in different ways. Heart disease is common among this population, and the patient's lung capacity lowers. Their metabolic rate decreases, leading to weight gain, and a decrease in muscle density affects the patient's mobility. Further illnesses and considerations will be covered later in the geriatric population section.

Psychologically, mental faculties may be starting to decline. However, this should not be assumed by the EMS provider. Patients at this age start to struggle with their decrease in independence, as they may have a caretaker, and should be treated with respect at all times.

Chapter Summary

Section "Planes and Perspectives"
- Anatomical planes are different ways to divide and view the body.
- You can use your understanding of these planes to help understand the placement of internal structures in relation to these planes and each other.

Section "Directional Terms"
- Position on the body is communicated using *directional terms*, which come in pairs and usually refer to one plane of the body.

Section "Positions"
- *Anatomical positions* refer to the position a body is in and can provide clinical clues of a patient's condition

Section "Major Skeletal Structures"
- The *skeletal system*, made up of bones and joints, serves many functions in the body, including the body's frame, providing structure and stability.
- Muscles attach to and form around this frame to allow for movement at the joints.
- The bones themselves have a few additional functions, such as the bone marrow-producing red blood cells.

Section "Human Development"
- As humans age, our bodies and minds develop and change.
- These physiological changes that natural development entails greatly affect human anatomy and how each age group responds to emergency situations, both physically and mentally.

Tricks of the Trade
- When trying to figure out which is the patient's left and right, just remember that your left is equal to the patient's right and vice versa.
- When trying to connect with children at a scene, don't be afraid to use a little humor or make a game for the child. For example, if the child is scared of the blood pressure cuff, equate it to a nice robot and try to make it fun.

Practice Questions
1. What directional term could be used to describe the position of a patient's knee in relation to their pelvic bone?

   (a) Ventral
   (b) Medial
   (c) Distal
   (d) Superficial

2. What is the order of the sections of the spinal vertebrae, starting from the top of the body and going down?

   (a) Lumbar, coccyx, sacral, thoracic, cervical
   (b) Cervical, thoracic, lumbar, sacral, coccyx
   (c) Cervical, thoracic, sacral, lumbar, coccyx
   (d) Thoracic, lumbar, cervical, sacral, coccyx

3. At what stage of human development will the provider have to be prepared to work closely with caretakers, due to a possible spike in separation anxiety?

   (a) Infant (0–1)
   (b) Toddler (1–3)
   (c) Preschooler (3–6)
   (d) School age (6–12)

4. What is the technical name for the commonly used recovery position?

   (a) Left lateral recumbent
   (b) Supine
   (c) Semi-Fowler
   (d) Fowler

Chapter 3
Fundamentals of Neurological Emergencies

Introduction

The human nervous system is arguably one of the most complex organ systems we are lucky enough to understand. Every thought, action, feeling, and sensation are the result of complex processing and communication between the brain, spinal cord, and other regions of the body.

In this chapter, you will begin to understand the physiology of the central and peripheral nervous system as well as the pathophysiology of common neurological illnesses. You will learn how to recognize a stroke, treat an actively seizing patient, and care for a patient with an altered mental status. This chapter will assist you in building your clinical intuition for suspecting neurological deficits and their overall implications in a medical emergency.

Overview of the Nervous System

3.1 Learning Objectives
Upon completing this section, you should be able to

- *understand* the role of the CNS and PNS,
- *identify* neuroanatomical structures and their functions,
- *infer* how the nervous system plays an overall role in health,
- *communicate* the difference between lateralization and localization.

Everything in the nervous system revolves around connections! Even a simple action such as turning a door knob, balancing a fall, or sending a text message is all thanks to highly coordinated neuronal interactions. Think about when you received an email congratulating you on your acceptance into an EMS program. You probably didn't realize the amount of neurological effort it took to process that information and the speed at which it was processed. You also might have not stopped to think about how that visual information was received by receptor cells, transmitted through the optic nerves, passed through the optic chiasm, and processed in the lateral geniculate nucleus, before being sent for continued processing in the occipital lobe. This is just a tiny example of the millions of neuronal interactions your brain coordinates simultaneously every second of every day.

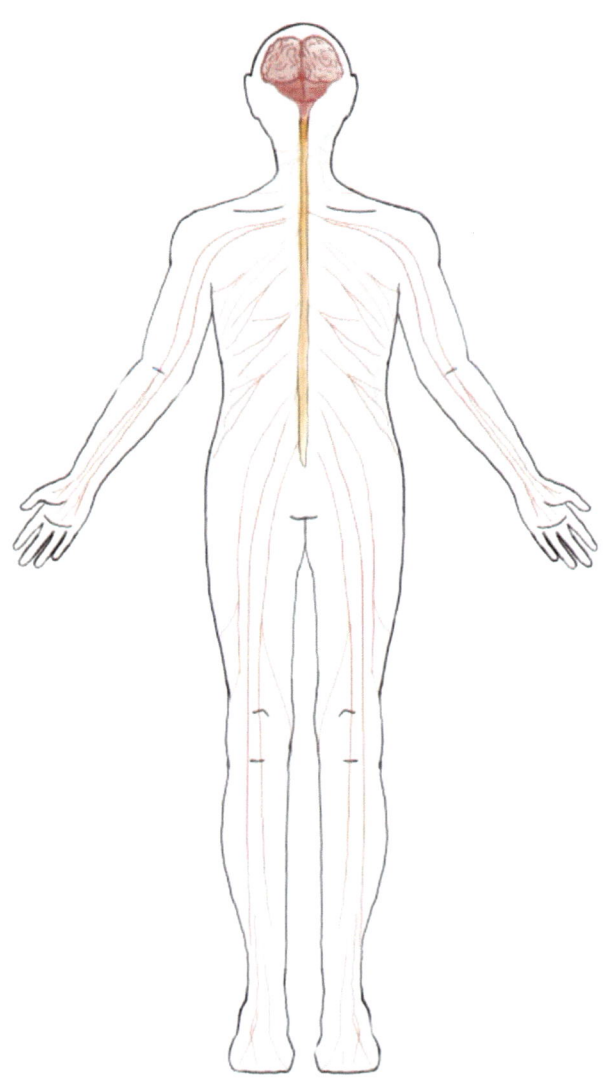

In medicine, when we talk about the nervous system, we're typically referring to a combination of both the *central nervous system* (*CNS*) and the *peripheral nervous system* (*PNS*). The CNS specifically refers to the brain and spinal cord duet, while the PNS is all other forms of neurological connections.

We can go on to further differentiate the nervous system into three subcategories:

- The *autonomic nervous system* is tasked with the coordination and execution of involuntary homeostatic tasks. For example, if you go out in chilly weather without a jacket, you'll probably shiver due to the brain's direction to rapidly contract and relax skeletal muscles, thus producing heat energy through respiration.
- The *enteric nervous system* is tasked with regulation of the digestive system, independent of the CNS. In some cases, this falls under the category of the autonomic nervous system.
- The *somatic nervous system* is tasked with voluntary motor control. Think of flipping the pages of this fancy textbook or swiping right on an app. This branch of the nervous system also covers automatic response, such as grabbing a stair handle if you accidentally miss a step.

The most relevant categorization of the nervous system for emergency providers is the *sympathetic nervous system* (colloquially known as "fight or flight") and the *parasympathetic nervous system* (also known as "rest and digest") which both fall under the autonomic nervous system. These systems collectively work to reach homeostasis through automatic regulation of heart rate, respiratory rate, and perspiration, among other internal and external actions. Let's say, for example, you come across your longtime crush. Your pupils may dilate, your liver may secrete epinephrine and norepinephrine, and your heart rate may go up. This is primarily due to the work of the sympathetic nervous system. On the other hand, right before you fall into a blissful rest in bed, your parasympathetic nervous system becomes activated. Your body temperature will come down, and so will your heart rate, and your body overall will be at rest.

Check Your Understanding: *The Nervous System*
You arrive on scene to treat a 47-year-old female for a suspected cardiac event. You are asked to comfort the patient's partner who is obviously anxious, sweating, and breathing rapidly. Which type of autonomic nervous system do you suspect is most dominant in the patient's partner?

The nervous system wouldn't be complete, of course, without neurons! *Neurons* make up one of three types of nerve cells, with the rest being *glial* cells and *myelin*.

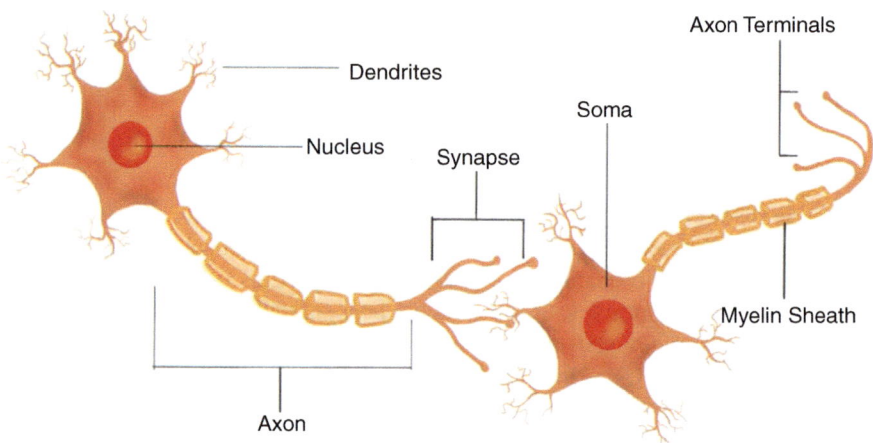

Neurons are major facilitators of information carried in *neurotransmitters* and are transmitted from a neuron to a target cell using electrical and chemical pathways. When a neuron sends a signal, we call it the *presynaptic* cell, whereas when a neuron receives it, we call it the *postsynaptic* cell. *Synapses* are regions where the presynaptic and postsynaptic cells meet, but do not physically touch, to conduct a transfer of information. Glial cells offer a support role to neurons by facilitating neuronal communication at the synapse, while myelin cells help insulate neurons to protect the integrity of transmitted electrical signals.

Whether or not a neuron will "fire" will depend on if an *action potential* is reached. An action potential indicates the likelihood of a neuron firing based upon the electrical charge of a neuron in the cell relative to outside the cell.

Check Your Understanding: *Nerve Cells*
When a seizure occurs, it is said that neurons are firing rapidly in an uncoordinated and inappropriate manner. Do you think that anti-seizure medications work to *increase* or *decrease* the action potential threshold? How do you know?

The *cerebrum* is what you might immediately imagine when you think of the brain. It is divided into two halves known as the right and left *hemispheres* connected by a structure called the *corpus callosum*. Within the cerebrum, there are four structures called *lobes* that correspond with particular functions. While it is true that we cannot simply say some parts of the brain are responsible for very specific functions, since lots of functions require integration from multiple parts of the brain, the term *localization* refers to the idea that specific structures of the brain carry out specific functions. The term *lateralization* refers to the idea that specific processes and functions are assigned to either the right or left hemisphere.

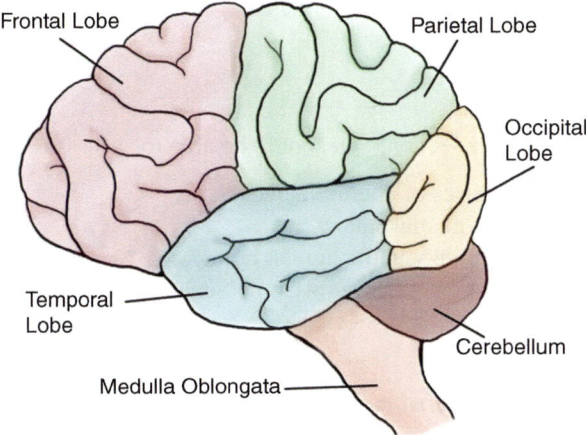

By now, scientists and psychologists have been able to correlate generalized functions with four lobes of the brain:

– The *frontal* lobe is implicated in personality traits and emotion, judgment, pre-execution of movement, and thought. It is also where *Broca's area* is found, the primary structure responsible for the production of speech.
– The *temporal* lobe is implicated in memory and is the home of *Wernicke's area*, the primary structure involved in the comprehension of language.
– The *parietal* lobe is implicated in perception of the world around us, involving body orientation and sensory discrimination.
– The *occipital* lobe is implicated in the receiving and processing of visual information.

Some other important structures to consider are those in the hindbrain:

– The *medulla oblongata*, or simply the medulla, assists in the regulation of involuntary life-sustaining actions such as respiratory rate and heart rate.
– The *cerebellum* is responsible for the facilitation of fine motor skills, coordination, and balance.

Around the cortex of the brain flows *cerebrospinal fluid* (*CSF*) which acts as a protective buffer and absorbs impact. We will discuss this at a greater depth later on in the chapter.

Check Your Understanding: *Lobes of the Brain*
You are assessing a suspected stroke patient who is unable to produce coherent speech. Which lobe of the brain is most likely afflicted?

Altered Mental Status

> **Learning Objectives**
> Upon completing this section, you should be able to
>
> - *understand* the causes of altered mental status,
> - *identify* a patient's mental status,
> - *infer* existing pathology in the human brain,
> - *communicate* a patient's Glasgow Coma Scale score.

We say a patient has an *altered mental status* (*AMS*) when some form of pathology causes a patient's behavior to seem inappropriate within a given context or setting.

Some common causes of AMS include the following:

- Alcohol and drugs
- Neurodegenerative disorders such as dementia
- Epilepsy
- Diabetic conditions
- Infection
- Metabolic disorders
- Hypoxia

Before we can understand a patient's level of alertness and orientation to the environment around them, we must first assess a patient's mental status using the AVPU scale.

> **Critical Skill:** *Using the AVPU Scale*
> - *Step 1:* As you walk into the patient's field of vision, do they immediately look at you? If so, they are considered "A" for alert. If not, proceed to Step 2.
> - *Step 2:* Try and communicate with your patient. Do they show any signs of responding to verbal stimuli such as eye opening or movement? If so, they are considered "V" for verbal. If not, proceed to Step 3.
> - *Step 3:* Perform a sternal rub, trapezius pinch, or other forms of painful stimuli in accordance with local protocols. Do they show any signs of responding to painful stimuli such as withdrawal from the stimulus? If so, they are considered "P" for pain. If not, proceed to Step 4.
> - *Step 4:* If the patient does not respond to any of these forms of stimuli, they are clinically considered "U" for unresponsiveness. Proceed accordingly.

After a level of mental status is understood and appropriately documented, we can now carefully assess the patient's alertness and orientation to the environment and situation.

Sometimes, providers may opt to use the *Glasgow Coma Scale* to assess a patient's *level of consciousness* (*LOC*) when pathology is suspected.

Critical Skill: *Assessing Alertness and Orientation*
This skill will assess a patient's alertness and orientation to time, location, and identity assuming the patient is conscious and no speech, language, or hearing barrier exists:

- *Step 1:* Ask the patient for their full name. Do they respond appropriately and accurately? If so, count this as 1 point.
- *Step 2:* Ask the patient if it is currently morning, afternoon, or night. Do they respond appropriately and accurately? If so, add 1 point.
- *Step 3:* Ask the patient what their current location is. Do they respond appropriately and accurately? If so, add 1 point.
- *Step 4:* Add up the total points and document your findings in terms of "A&O." For example, if they answer all your questions appropriately, you can deem this patient "A&OX3," denoting the patient is alert and oriented tested three times. This is read as "A and O times 3" when corresponding with other medical professionals. If the patient answers all questions inappropriately, they are considered disoriented.

Glasgow Coma Scale		
Eye Opening Response	Spontaneous--open with blinking at baseline	4
	To verbal stimuli, command, speech 3 points	3
	To pain only (not applied to face) 2 points	2
	No response	1
Verbal Response	Oriented	5
	Confused conversation, but able to answer questions	4
	Inappropriate words	3
	Incomprehensible speech	2
	No response	1
Motor Response	Obeys commands for movement	6
	Purposeful movement to painful stimulus	5
	Withdraws in response to pain	4
	Flexion in response to pain (decorticate posturing)	3
	Extension response in response to pain (decerebrate posturing)	2
	No response	1

Check Your Understanding: *Assessing Mental Status*
You arrive at the scene of a 57-year-old patient who is the victim of suspected domestic violence. Upon your thorough questioning, it becomes evident that the patient is aware of their location, but not their identity or the time of day. What would you rate this patient on a scale of disoriented to A&OX3?

Traumatic Brain Injuries

Learning Objectives
Upon completing this section, you should be able to

- *understand* mechanisms of injury for TBIs,
- *identify* a suspected TBI,
- *infer* the existence of a suspected brain bleed,
- *communicate* appropriate care post concussion.

Picture this: You opened up the top cabinet in a kitchen and reached down to grab something from the bottom drawer, and then as soon as you stand up, you meet the misfortune of hitting your head on the open cabinet. You might be feeling dizzy, irritated, or even nauseous after. This is called a *traumatic brain injury (TBI)*. We say that a patient has experienced a TBI when a direct or indirect force causes acute neurological symptoms in a patient.

Injury occurs when potential energy is transferred to the human body in a way that damages tissue. To express this in terms of physics, we say that potential energy $= (0.5)(mass)(velocity)^2$, meaning that the greatest indicator of severity of injury is the velocity (or speed) of the force.

Common mechanisms of injury for TBIs include the following:

- Motor vehicle collisions
- Pedestrian struck by a motor vehicle
- Domestic assault

As your intuition would probably tell you, the more severe the mechanism of injury, the more severe the TBI. It is important to consider that TBIs vary from concussion-type injuries to brain bleeds.

If there was a loss of consciousness associated with a TBI, we would call this "positive LOC" and denote this as *(+) LOC*, whereas intuitively, *(−) LOC* would imply there was no reported loss of consciousness.

Concussion is a type of TBI that is often called an invisible injury, because standard neuroimaging techniques such as MRIs and CT scans cannot detect the presence or absence of a concussion. Concussion is primarily diagnosed by a healthcare provider based upon neurological exam and self-reported symptomatology. Concussion symptoms typically do not appear until days to weeks after impact, usually with a recovery period of weeks to months depending on the severity of the mechanism of injury.

Signs and Symptoms of Concussion
- Sleeping issues
- Irritability
- Emotional/behavioral issues
- Photophobia and/or phonophobia
- Nausea with or without vomiting
- Loss of consciousness

An old yet popular myth of concussion that was infamous among parents with young children was to advise parents not to let their child sleep for 24 hours if they suspected a concussion or it would develop into a brain bleed. This is incredibly untrue; in fact, the recommended treatment for concussion is cognitive rest. Patients are also advised to refrain from the use of electronics, decrease screen time, avoid operating machinery, and avoid unnecessary activity. Concussions typically resolve on their own.

Check Your Understanding: *Concussions*
You are responding to the scene of a motor vehicle collision where a car collided into a telephone pole. Which of the following is the greatest indicator of the severity of a suspected TBI?

(a) Mass of the vehicle
(b) Mass of the telephone pole
(c) Speed of the vehicle
(d) Age of the driver

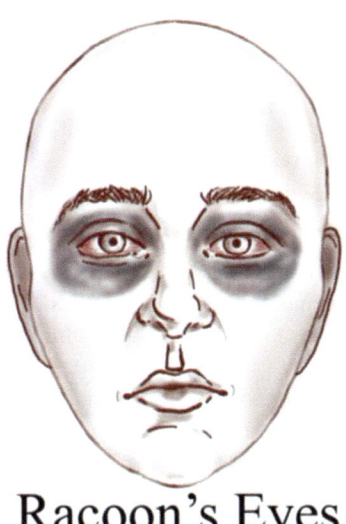

Racoon's Eyes

Brain bleeds (*intracerebral hemorrhages*) are a type of TBI that is often associated with greater morbidity and mortality and is typically indicative of a more severe mechanism of injury. Common signs of brain bleeds include *racoon's eyes* and *battle's sign*.

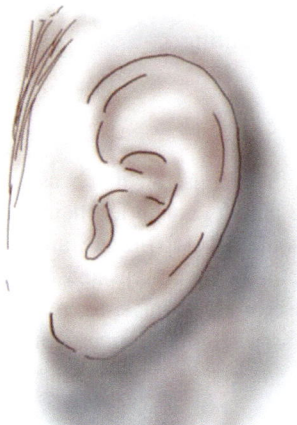

Battle Signs

At this juncture, we are already familiar that cerebrospinal fluid surrounds the brain tissue in the skull.

We need to remember that the skull is a closed system, meaning that if we increase pressure on one side of the system, it will increase pressure everywhere. Under this assumption, we can understand how the growth of a tumor or bleeding in the brain can increase pressure everywhere in the skull. We call this pressure *intracranial pressure* (*ICP*), and through a diagnostic test called *Cushing's triad,* we can suspect if ICP is increased.

Cushing's triad is defined as follows:

– An increase in systolic blood pressure
– A slow heart rate
– A slow respiratory rate

It is important to consider that these vital signs may be present in patients without increased ICP and that patients may have pupil abnormalities due to another underlying medical condition. As providers, we cannot base our clinical impression on one test, sign, or symptom—but based upon a collection of clinical evidence combined with probable cause. Good intuition and common sense are prerequisite to practicing good emergency medicine.

Check Your Understanding: *Cushing's Triad*
You are arriving at the scene of a patient who was ejected from a motorcycle and was not wearing a helmet. Which combination of vital signs might make you suspect an intracerebral hemorrhage?

(a) HR: 56 BPM; BP: 156/88 mmHg; RR: 8 RPM
(b) HR: 104 BPM; BP: 124/80 mmHg; RR: 16 RPM
(c) HR: 54 BPM; BP: 90/60 mmHg; RR: 14 RPM
(d) HR: 116 BPM; BP: 88/76 mmHg; RR: 8 RPM

Cerebrovascular Accidents

Learning Objectives
Upon completing this section, you should be able to

- *understand* risk factors of stroke,
- *identify* a suspected stroke,
- *infer* on the region of existing pathology,
- *communicate* a "Code Stroke" to the receiving treatment facility.

Picture this: You are driving to the grocery store with a friend when she suddenly complains of a headache. You ask her what's wrong, but she replies with words that are barely discernible. You notice her right arm leaves the steering wheel. Something is not right. You recall studying about cerebrovascular accidents in your EMS course and recognize that she is exhibiting signs of a stroke, so you act quickly and safely bring the vehicle to a stop and call 911.

Cerebrovascular accidents (*CVAs*), also known as strokes, are a condition in which the brain tissue is deprived of oxygen-rich blood. When this occurs, blood flow to the brain tissue is disrupted, and brain damage results.

Early recognition of strokes is paramount to proper care as this will dictate interventions performed in the field as well as transport decisions. Patients often benefit from transport to specialized facilities dedicated to stroke care. Risk factors of strokes include hypertension, diabetes, atrial fibrillation, and usage of tobacco products, and even genetic factors are involved.

At this level, we are mostly concerned with two types of stroke, ischemic and hemorrhagic.

Ischemic strokes account for approximately 90% of all strokes and occur when a clot is occluding an artery that supplies oxygen-rich blood to brain tissue. *Hemorrhagic* strokes account for the remaining 10% and are often secondary to trauma or *aneurysm*.

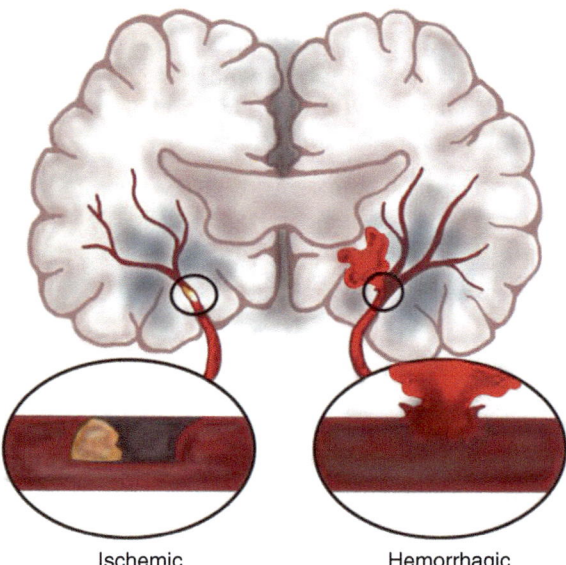

Ischemic   Hemorrhagic

In the hemorrhagic stroke secondary to an aneurysm story, a region of the wall of an artery within the skull begins to weaken due to a genetic mutation. Because the vessel wall is very elastic, blood starts to collect and pool into the weakened area, creating a balloon-like structure known as the aneurysm. Over time, the aneurysm becomes so massive that it bursts. Two major issues are occurring here:

I. Old stagnant blood that previously pooled in the aneurysm is now exposed to brain tissue, which is toxic.
II. There is now a rip in the artery, so blood is diverted to a different pathway than intended.

Treatment of a CVA focuses on supportive care and rapid transport. Although it may appear that little intervention can be done from the role of an EMS provider, there are many steps that can be taken to assist the patient in attaining a positive outcome. This includes assuring the airway is open and patent, breathing is adequate, and circulation of blood in the body is maintained. Vital signs should be taken, including pulse rate, blood pressure, oxygen saturation (SPO2%), lung sounds, and blood glucose levels. In patients exhibiting signs and symptoms of hypoxia, oxygen therapy should be initiated. Do **not** delay transport to a treatment facility.

Critical Skill: *Stroke Assessment*
This skill will assess for signs and symptoms of CVA. Presence of any of the following signs should lead to a high index of suspicion for CVA:

- *Step 1:* Ask the patient to smile for you or to show you their teeth. Monitor for unilateral facial drooping.

- *Step 2:* Instruct the patient to close their eyes and then raise the patient's arms in front of them. Be sure to support their hands. Release their hands, and check for signs of arm drift for at least ten seconds.
- *Step 3:* Ask the patient to repeat back to you a simple phrase. Popular phrases used by emergency physicians and neurologists include "Today is a sunny day" and "You can't teach an old dog new tricks." Listen for any speech abnormalities including slurred speech, inappropriate words, or delayed response.
- *Step 4:* If any of the above signs or symptoms occur, record your observations, and prepare for rapid transport.

Sometimes, a patient may present with stroke-like symptoms that resolve on their own. This is known as a *transient ischemic attack* (*TIA*) or a mini-stroke and is often a warning sign that a more severe stroke is on the way. Continue to treat this patient as a Code Stroke, and alert the receiving facility immediately.

Seizures

Learning Objectives
Upon completing this section, you should be able to

- *understand* the condition of epilepsy and other seizure disorders,
- *identify* signs and symptoms of a seizure,
- *infer* causes of a seizure,
- *communicate* to a patient in a postictal state.

You are called to respond to the scene of an adult female convulsing. Upon arrival, her spouse tells you that she briefly smelt an odd scent before collapsing. You recognize this to be a generalized tonic-clonic seizure.

Seizures are neuropathological phenomena in which there is a disruption in the normal electrical activity of the brain which results in convulsions or other abnormal neurological presentations. There are many types of seizures that exist; however, we are most concerned with two major classes, *focal* seizures and *generalized tonic-clonic* (*GTC*) *seizures*:

- Focal seizures (also known as "petit mal" seizures) traditionally start in one region of the brain and may spread with varying severity.
- Generalized tonic-clonic seizures (also known as "grand mal" seizures) result in diffuse involvement of the right and left brain hemispheres.

Stages of a Generalized Tonic-Clonic Seizure
1. *Aura*: The aura phase is an accurate indicator that a seizure is about to occur, and patients diagnosed with seizure disorders are typically aware of what their auras are. An aura can be a sudden sensation or feeling such as an odd taste and sweet smell, a high pitch sound, or a sudden sense of doom. Not all seizures are preceded by an aura, although most are.
2. *Tonic or atonic*: In the second phase of a grand mal seizure, patients typically experience either brief muscle stiffness (tonic) or a complete loss of muscle tone (atonic). Some patients may experience their head turning to one side.
3. *Clonic*: The clonic phase is characterized as the rapid relaxation and contraction of muscles. This phase is when the convulsions occur.
4. *Postictal*: The postictal state constitutes the recovery phase of the seizure. The patient may be fatigued, disoriented, and in some cases combative.

Critical Skill: *Responding to a GTC Seizure*
- *Step 1:* If the patient is standing, assist them to the floor to avoid injury from fall.
- *Step 2:* Place the patient on their left side. This is known as the recovery position. This will mitigate the risk of aspiration should the patient vomit. Be sure to take note of the time of onset of the seizure.

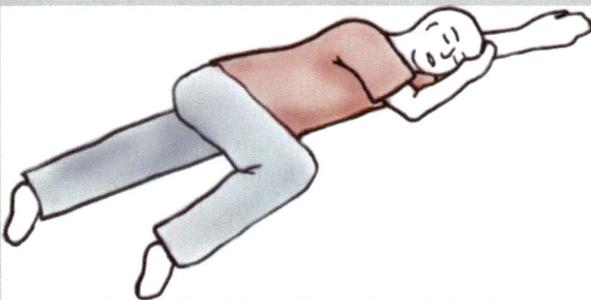

- *Step 3:* Remove any obstructions, such as furniture, from the vicinity of the patient.
- *Step 4:* Support the head with a pillow or other soft material
- *Step 5:* Loosen any tight-fitting clothing and remove ties, hats, glasses, etc.
- *Step 6:* If the patient exhibits signs or symptoms of hypoxia, initiate oxygen therapy according to local protocols.

- *Step 7:* If the seizure lasts longer than 3 minutes, consider immediate transport as the patient may be experiencing status epilepticus.
  Note: Do **not** place anything into the mouth of the patient. Contrary to popular belief, patients are not capable of swallowing their tongue. Although the tongue can fall to the back of the oropharynx, resulting in obstruction, this can be corrected through the application of the head-tilt/chin-lift procedure following the cessation of the seizure activity.
  An appropriate history should be gathered from family or bystanders, focusing specifically on possible history of seizures and duration of the seizure.

Immediate priority transport should be considered for seizure patients who

- hurt themselves or hurt others,
- are pregnant,
- are diabetic,
- have a seizure lasting longer than 3–5 minutes (this could indicate status epilepticus),
- have seizure for the first time.

Chapter Summary

Section "Overview of the Nervous System"
- The *central nervous system* (*CNS*) specifically refers to the brain and spinal cord, while the *peripheral nervous system* (*PNS*) is all other forms of neurological connections.
- *Localization* refers to the idea that specific structures of the brain carry out specific functions. *Lateralization* refers to the idea that specific processes and functions are assigned to a specific hemisphere.

Section "Altered Mental Status"
- *Altered mental status* (*AMS*) occurs when some form of pathology causes a patient's behavior to seem inappropriate within a given context or setting and can be the result of an underlying phenomenon such as alcohol/drug use, a neurodegenerative illness, or a metabolic disorder.
- The *Glasgow Coma Scale* and the *AVPU* scale are methods of assessing a patient's mental status and level of consciousness rapidly.

Section "Traumatic Brain Injuries"
- *Traumatic brain injury* (*TBI*) occurs when a direct or indirect force causes acute neurological symptoms in a patient. Concussion and intracerebral hemorrhage are types of TBIs.

- *Cushing's triad*, *racoon's eyes*, and *Battle's sign* are all signs of a suspected brain bleed.

Section "Cerebrovascular Accidents"

- *Cerebrovascular accidents* (*CVAs*), or strokes, occur when brain tissue is deprived of oxygen-rich blood. The two types of stroke are *ischemic* and *hemorrhagic.*
- *Transient ischemic attacks* (*TIAs*) are mini-strokes and should be treated and assessed just like all other types of stroke

Section "Seizures"

- *Seizures* are neuropathological phenomena in which there is a disruption in the normal electrical activity of the brain which results in abnormal neurological presentations.
- Immediate priority transport should be considered for patients that meet high-risk criteria.

Practice Questions

1. What is the final stage in a GTC seizure?

    (a) Tonic
    (b) Clonic
    (c) Postictal
    (d) Aura

2. While performing a basic neurological assessment, your patient can tell you their name and the time of day, but not where they are or what events led up to your arrival. How would this patient be rated in terms of alertness and orientation?

    (a) A&O × 3
    (b) A&O × 1
    (c) A&O × 2
    (d) A&O × 4

3. You arrive on scene to a 55-year-old patient. When trying to communicate with them, you notice that their speech is slurred and the left side of their face is drooping. Upon further assessment, you note that the patient cannot keep one of their arms steadily held in front of them. Which neurological emergency is indicated?

   (a) Traumatic brain injury
   (b) Absence seizure
   (c) Overdose
   (d) Cerebrovascular accident

4. What is true about a concussion?

   (a) It is caused by bleeding in the brain.
   (b) It is considered an "invisible injury" because it does not show up on MRIs.
   (c) A patient with a concussion should not fall asleep.
   (d) It is a life-threatening emergency.

Chapter 4
Head, Neck, and Spinal Injuries

Introduction

As we have previously learned, one of the most crucial networks of the human body is the central nervous system, protected by the skull and spine. These protective measures are often successful at their jobs. However, any system failure that compromises the integrity of the head, neck, and spine could lead to grave consequences ranging from loss of sensation to paralysis or even death. We will discuss specific types of these injuries in this chapter.

As a first responder, you must be able to identify situations where there is an increased likelihood of skull or spinal damage and take the proper precautions to stop any further damage from occurring. There are many skills in your toolbox which can be used to help care for a patient with a head, neck, or spinal injury.

Overview of Head, Neck, and Spinal Anatomy and Injures

Learning Objectives
Upon completing this section, you should be able to

- *understand* the effects of injuries to the head, neck, or spine;
- *identify* if an injury is potentially life-threatening;
- *infer* possible internal injuries that may be present;
- *communicate* priority concerns at the BLS level.

There are various anatomical structures which make up the head, neck, and spine due to the many different possible types of injuries that can occur.

© The Author(s), under exclusive license to Springer Nature Switzerland AG 2021
C. Ventura et al., *The Emergency Medical Responder*,
https://doi.org/10.1007/978-3-030-64396-6_4

The Scalp

The outer layer of the head is the *scalp* which is made up of skin as well as a layer of dense connective tissue. These structures do have quite a bit of surface vascularity and can easily be damaged. Even slight damage to the scalp can have a relatively high amount of bleeding, but often this bleeding will not be life-threatening. Keep any scalp bleeding in mind, but do not let it distract you from any serious life threats. Scalp bleeds should be treated like most other bleeds, with direct pressure. When assessing the scalp, be sure to perform a manual sweep of the head with your gloves as hair may hide any bleeds or other injuries. Check the front and back of your gloves routinely to check for any noticeable blood.

The Skull

Below the scalp, we have the bony portion of the head known as the skull or *cranium*, which serves as the main protective layer of the head. Injuries to the skull are very severe but not always life-threatening. If the brain is exposed, place a dressing on the damaged area, and transport to the appropriate facility. The dressing must be placed loosely to allow for any swelling of the brain. In the case of an injury to the head of a patient wearing a helmet, do not remove the helmet as it may be holding any loose segments of the cranium in place. Helmets may only be removed if it improves treatments of any life threats or spinal stabilization.

Dura and Arachnoid Mater

Below the cranium, there are two protective membranes which include the *dura mater* and the *arachnoid mater*. These are areas below the subdural space and the subarachnoid space. Even if there is no visible bleeding or damage to the scalp or cranium, there could still be internal damage beneath. The main concern of internal bleeding is the increased pressure on the brain as blood fills these spaces below the membranes. This is known as *increased intracranial pressure* (increased ICP), which is often indicated by Cushing's triad. The skull is a closed system, unlike the abdomen which can extend to create more available space. This means that if pressure increases due to subdural or subarachnoid bleeding, pressure increases everywhere in the CNS. This pressure can cause neurological deficits or even cellular death within the brain.

If you suspect any trauma to the head, you should perform a brief neurological assessment and assess vital signs for Cushing's triad. A Glasgow Coma Score and AVPU scale score should be documented, and any changes in these values should be documented too. The highest priority at the BLS level is to maintain a patent airway to support adequate respiration, ventilation, and oxygenation.

The *spinal column* is a set of 33 vertebrae which extend the length of the trunk of the body from the base of the skull. As discussed in Chap. 2, the spinal cord is made up of five sections: cervical, thoracic, lumbar, sacral, and coccygeal. You can remember this as "Can't think like susan can" or, my favorite, "Christmas time lives Santa Clause." As neural impulses travel from the brain down, damage to a region will often affect all sections below it. We can thus approximate where the injury is located as sensation will not be present below the injury. When there is a possible injury to the spinal column, it is critical that spinal stabilization is applied.

Check Your Understanding: *Head Injuries*
Which of the following scenarios would most likely be the most immediately life-threatening to a patient:

(a) External hemorrhage from a scalp laceration
(b) Internal hemorrhage in the subdural space due to a fall
(c) A missing segment of the skull from a blunt weapon attack
(d) Damage to the lumbar spinal cord in a car collision

Identification of Possible Spinal Injuries

Learning Objectives
Upon completing this section, you should be able to

- *understand* how mechanism of injury affects the severity of injury,
- *identify* the affected location of different spinal injuries,
- *infer* types of spinal injury,
- *communicate* when spinal stabilization is necessary.

Because most spinal injuries are internal, we must learn to be able to use secondary information to determine the presence of any spinal injuries. This includes the assessment of other areas and systems of the body and thorough consideration of the mechanism of injury. Before we discuss specific effects of spinal injuries, we must first recognize the types of injuries that can occur to the spinal cord. Each type of injury is categorized by the direction of the force and whether it involves the vertebral body, the vertebral arch, or both.

Compression Injury
In this type of injury, a force is applied downward in the lengthwise direction of the spine. This force is distributed through the vertebrae, but in some cases, the force causes one or more of the vertebrae to be crushed and fractured. The vertebral body is primarily damaged. This is typically seen in fall victims who land head first, such as in diving accidents.

Hyperextension Injury
This injury occurs when there is a force applied parallel to the spinal cord from the front of the patient causing the neck to bend back too far. This in turn causes the vertebral arch to be compressed and fractured. An example of this is whiplash from a car collision.

Flexion Injury

In flexion injuries, force is applied to the front which causes the vertebrae to shift forward and separate or dislocate from the remainder of the spinal cord. In this case, the vertebrae itself will often remain intact. When a rotational force is introduced to this situation, it can be called a flexion-rotation injury. This injury has become popular in movies when the enemies are killed by twisting their neck quickly. While probably not the most effective due to the force required to perform the kill, it does indeed look cool.

Distraction Injury

Distraction injuries occur when a pulling force is applied to a portion of the spinal column causing separation of two vertebrae.

Penetration Injury

Exactly as it sounds, penetration injuries occur when any external force causes penetration to a region of the spinal column.

We can now start to think about what mechanisms of injury would cause these injuries. A good rule of thumb is to think about great forces applied to the patient, such as motor vehicle collisions or blunt weapon injuries to the back. The most common mechanism of injury is falls from greater than three times the patient's height. You should still keep in mind that shorter heights may cause spinal injuries in elderly patients or with focused points of impacts such as in a flight of stairs.

Even though we can use this knowledge of the mechanism to initially predict if there will be a spinal injury, we want to also consider the signs and symptoms of the patient. The higher in the spinal cord the injury is, the more of the body will be affected. In general, we are primarily worried about paralysis of the patient, and thus, we will want to assess the pulse motor and sensory status of the patient religiously.

Assessing Circulation, Motor, and Sensory (CMS) Distal Function

CMS distal function should be checked in your secondary assessment, before and after splinting, and routinely en route if transportation to a receiving facility is abnormally long:

- To assess for circulation, check for a distal pulse such as a pedal or radial pulse. Check for capillary refill; does it exceed 3 seconds? Check for temperature and color. Is there localized cyanosis, and is the skin cold?
- To assess for motor function, ask the patient to wiggle their toes and/or fingers. Are they able to do so? Is there a restricted range of motion?
- To assess for sensory function, touch a patient's finger/toe, and ask them to correctly identify the digit. Is sensation intact? Can the patient proprioceptively identify the location of their digits?

In cases of major injury to the spinal cord, a *priapism*, a painful persistent erection of the penis due to a head injury, or incontinence may occur. Check for a priapism using the back of your gloved hand. It is also important that you assess for any physical deformities to the spine as well. Paralysis is what we are primarily trying to avoid. Damage to the upper areas of the spinal cord, such as the cervical spine region, can have much more life-threatening effects on life-sustaining functions, such as the respiratory system. It is also still important to not neglect continual assessment and management of the patient's airway, breathing, and circulation. Again, airway management is one of your highest priorities. Specific interventions at the BLS level will comprise spinal stabilization, immobilization, and transport which we will discuss further in the next section.

Check Your Understanding: *Spinal Injuries*
You are called to the scene of a patient who has been assaulted and stabbed in the spine with a knife. You stabilize the knife and provide immediate transport while managing airway, breathing, and circulation of the patient. Which type of spinal injury does this patient likely have?

(a) Compression injury
(b) Penetrating injury
(c) Hyperextension injury
(d) Distraction injury

Methods for Head and Spinal Stabilization

Learning Objectives
Upon completing this section, you should be able to

* *understand* the placement of various spinal stabilization devices,
* *identify* which spinal stabilization method is indicated,
* *infer* the efficacy of different spinal stabilization methods,
* *communicate* to a patient what to do in a suspected spinal injury.

As you have now learned, there are many possible ways in which a patient can sustain an injury to their skull or spinal cord, and rapid intervention is important. There is a high likelihood of lifelong complications if the proper precautions are not taken. At the BLS level, the management for head and spinal injuries can be simplified to immobilization of the affected area. In almost all cases of suspected head/spinal injury, you should never move the patient's head until you provide some form of spinal stabilization, such as the application of a cervical collar. When approaching the patient, always approach toward the front. If you approach from the back or side of the patient, they will have a tendency to look and move toward you, possibly resulting in severe injury.

Manual Stabilization
Our first line of care for any possible head, neck, or spinal injury is manual stabilization. Manual stabilization is the most basic form of cervical spine stabilization in

which the neck and head are supported and held in by the hands of the first responder. In performing this supportive care, it is important to take into consideration the positioning of your patient. If the patient is standing or sitting, manual stabilization will consist of the first responder placing their hands on the shoulders with their palms providing support to the neck and extension of the thumbs to provide support to the head. An alternative method is placement of the palms on the sides of the head with fingers splayed to provide greater range of support. If the patient is standing, we want to place them in a more stable supine position by performing what is known as a standing takedown. In this maneuver, a backboard is placed behind the patient, and the patient is gradually lowered, while your partner supports the bottom of the blackboard to prevent slippage. This maneuver is only to be done after the placement of a more permanent method of cervical spine stabilization.

If the patient is sitting, additional methods can be used to stabilize the patient which will be discussed at a later point. If the patient is already in a supine position, manual stabilization can be done by the first responder holding the patient's shoulders and providing support to the head and neck with the forearms. It is key that when any form of manual stabilization is performed, the first responder's hands remain firm and rigid. Manual stabilization is the least effective method of spinal stabilization as it only covers the cervical spine, and it is very difficult in practice for the first responder to maintain the rigid hand placement for long periods. With that said, this form of spinal stabilization is only temporary till more effective forms of stabilization can be implemented.

Cervical Collar Use

A more effective and secure method for stabilization of the cervical spine is the placement of a cervical collar. A *cervical collar* (*C-collar*) is a rigid device which is placed around the neck of a patient which inhibits movement of the head and cervical spine, providing stabilization and alignment. This is to be placed as soon as possible in a patient with a suspected spinal injury. Once the C-collar is placed, it is not to be removed unless you are directed to by a physician.

Critical Skill: *Placement of a Cervical Collar*
- *Step 1:* Provide manual cervical spine stabilization.
- *Step 2:* Measure the approximate size of the patient's neck with placement of one's fingers along the neck.
- *Step 3:* Select the appropriate-size C-collar, or adjust if using a variable-size C-collar.
- *Step 4:* Slide cervical collar under the neck of the patient to the appropriate position, and flip up chin rest if applicable.
- *Step 5:* Wrap both sides of the collar around the neck of the patient and secure appropriately.

As the methods we have discussed to this point have only been for stabilization of the cervical spine, we will need other tools to manage possible injuries of the other areas of the spine. The most common piece of equipment for spinal stabilization other than the C-collar is the long backboard. A *long backboard* is a flat board made of rigid material such as a polymer used to lift and move a patient while maintaining the patient's spine in a neutral position. The long backboard is used in conjunction with straps and head blocks to secure the patient. If there is suspicion of a major spinal injury, a long backboard may be used. When moving the patient onto the backboard, it is of great importance that you roll the patient as a unit so as to not cause any additional spinal injuries. If the patient must be adjusted while on the backboard, it must be done with motions in alignment with the spinal cord. The patient should be placed on the backboard supine with arms across the body in a hugging position.

Critical Skill: *Placement of a Long Backboard*
- *Step 1:* Position the patient in supine position and provide manual stabilization.
- *Step 2:* Assess for pulse motor and sensory status in all extremities.
- *Step 3:* Properly place a C-collar on the patient.
- *Step 4:* Roll the patient on the long backboard.
- *Step 5:* Secure the patient to the long backboard using strap.
- *Step 6:* Place head blocks on the patient.
- *Step 7:* Reassess pulse motor and sensory status in all extremities.
  Note: Whenever a patient with cervical spine precautions is moved, it must be done in accordance with direction of the person holding the patient's head. This is colloquially known as "on the head's count." This is done to prevent uncoordinated movements of team members from further injuring the patient.

Another common variation of the long blackboard is the short backboard. It is used if the patient is in an obstructed sitting position and is used in the same manner as the long backboard. An alternative to the short backboard is the Kendrick Extrication Device (KED), which can be used for vehicle extractions where a spinal injury is likely. Once the patient is secured with the KED, they will be placed on a long backboard.

Critical Skill: *Placement of a Kendrick Extrication Device*
- *Step 1:* Position the patient in supine position and provide manual stabilization.
- *Step 2:* Assess for pulse motor and sensory status in all extremities.
- *Step 3:* Properly place a C-collar on the patient.

- *Step 4:* Slide KED behind the patient's back.
- *Step 5:* Apply the torso straps to the patient in order of yellow, red, and then green.
- *Step 6:* Apply black leg straps to the patient.
- *Step 7:* Secure the patient's head to KED.
- *Step 8:* Tighten straps in the same order as they were secured.
- *Step 9:* Move the patient to a long backboard.

As we have learned, there are many different types of devices which can be used to provide spinal stabilization to a trauma patient—any of which can be used in conjunction with each other. It is important to be able to identify which scenario calls for which device. Regardless of whichever device is used, it is best to minimize any unnecessary patient movement.

Check Your Understanding: Spinal Stabilization
You are called to respond to an unconscious male who has fallen from a two-story building. The patient is unresponsive and is currently in a prone position. It is suspected that a spinal injury may be present. Which method of spinal stabilization is **not** indicated at any point in this situation?

(a) Kendrick Extrication Device
(b) Long backboard
(c) Cervical spine collar
(d) Manual spinal stabilization

It is important to note that there has been much recent evidence to encourage against the use of backboard immobilization and KEDs, as it may do more harm to the patient than good. Many local and state protocols have begun to shift away from the regular use of backboarding, even when spinal injuries are present. Always consult your instructor, medical director, or education officer to verify approved precautionary protocols. The use of backboards and KEDs still remains part of the national standards.

Chapter Summary

Section "Overview of Head, Neck, and Spinal Anatomy and Injures"
- The scalp, the top layer of the head, will bleed with slight trauma but is often not immediately life-threatening.
- The cranium is the bony portion of the head. If there is an exposed area, loosely cover it with a moist dressing.

- Internal bleeding may occur in the subdural and subarachnoid layers, ultimately causing pressure on the brain and, in turn, neurological deficits.
- The spinal cord is made up of five sections, and injuries can easily cause paralysis to the area injured as well as any lower areas.

Section "Identification of Possible Spinal Injuries"
- Injuries to the spine are classified by the direction of the force applied as well as the part of the spinal cord that is affected.
- Mechanisms of injury can be used to predict if a spinal injury is present as well as the type of injury.
- In patients that may have a spinal injury, assessment of circulatory, motor, and sensory status is critically important. It is also crucial to note the presence of a priapism, incontinence, tingling, or respiratory/cardiac dysfunction.

Section "Methods for Head and Spinal Stabilization"
- In a patient suspected to have a spinal injury, it is of great importance to provide spinal stabilization using temporary manual stabilization and stabilization devices such as a long backboard or C-collar.

Practice Questions
1. You arrive at a car crash, where one vehicle has been hit head on by another. One of the drivers in the collision starts to complain of neck pain. What kind of spinal injury can you suspect?

    (a) Flexion injury
    (b) Hyperextension injury
    (c) Distraction injury
    (d) Compression injury

2. When assessing a patient for spinal injuries, you notice a deformation in the patient's neck. What section of the spine does that deformation most likely lie on?

    (a) Cervical
    (b) Thoracic
    (c) Lumbar
    (d) Sacrum

3. What is always the final step when backboarding?

    (a) Making sure the straps are tight
    (b) Lifting the board into a transport vehicle
    (c) Reassessing sensory motor function in all extremities
    (d) Placing and cervical spine collar

Chapter 5
Airway and Cardiothoracic Emergencies

Introduction

Airway, breathing, and circulation are the crux of good emergency medical care. We say that without a patent airway, we have impaired breathing and, inevitably, impaired circulation. Maintenance of ABCs comprises the EMS clinician's most critical priority.

This chapter will provide an overview of the anatomy of the upper and lower airway, as well as the structures within the thoracic cavity. We will also discuss how to identify common cardiac- and respiratory-related emergencies and how to treat them at the BLS level.

Airway and Cardiothoracic Anatomy

Learning Objectives
Upon completing this section, you should be able to

- *understand* what is within the thoracic cavity,
- *identify* the structures of the upper and lower airways,
- *infer* the mechanism of the heart,
- *communicate* the purpose of the system within the thoracic cavity.

The thoracic cavity makes up the upper half of our torso and is home to some of the most vital organs in our bodies. The structures in the thoracic cavity can be organized into three categories, cardiac structures, respiratory structures, and the skeletal structures formed to protect the whole system.

© The Author(s), under exclusive license to Springer Nature
Switzerland AG 2021
C. Ventura et al., *The Emergency Medical Responder*,
https://doi.org/10.1007/978-3-030-64396-6_5

The skeletal structure that surrounds the thoracic cavity is the *rib cage*. This was already mentioned briefly when we discussed skeletal structures in Chap. 2, but just to review, the rib cage is made up of individual ribs that attach to the sternum and is meant to protect the vital organs in the thoracic cavity.

The core of the cardiac system also lies within the thoracic cavity.

The *heart* is the organ that pumps blood throughout the body and lies left of the sternum. It is split into four chambers, two atria and two ventricles. Deoxygenated blood is pumped from the body, through the right atria and ventricle, and then to the lungs to reabsorb oxygen. Then, the blood is pumped from the lungs, to the left atria and ventricle, then back to the body to deliver oxygen. The heart pumps blood by contracting and relaxing, which occur because of an electrical signal sent through the heart.

The *aorta* is a large artery through which oxygenated blood travels from the left ventricle to the rest of the body.

The *inferior and superior vena cava* are the veins that deoxygenated blood uses to travel from the body to the right atria.

There are other vessels that connect the heart with the lungs and deliver blood to the heart muscle, and vessels that carry blood throughout the rest of the body will be discussed later.

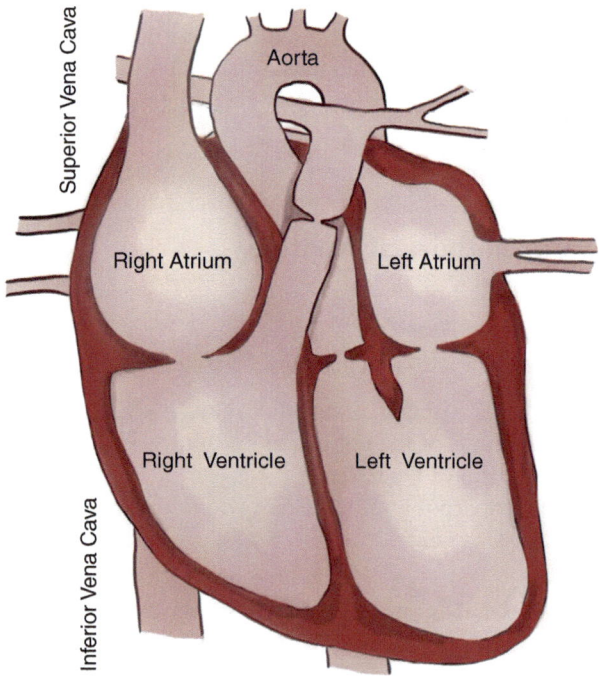

Another system which has its core in the thoracic cavity is the respiratory system. This includes all structures needed for respiration and can be split into the upper and lower airways.

Upper Airway

The *nasopharynx* and *oropharynx* are the cavities within the nose and mouth through which air and oxygen enter the body and carbon dioxide is expelled.

The *pharynx* is where the nasopharynx and oropharynx converge.

The *epiglottis* is a movable flap which separates the trachea and the esophagus, ensuring the air does not enter the stomach and solids do not enter the lungs.

The *larynx* lies under the epiglottis and leads into the trachea.

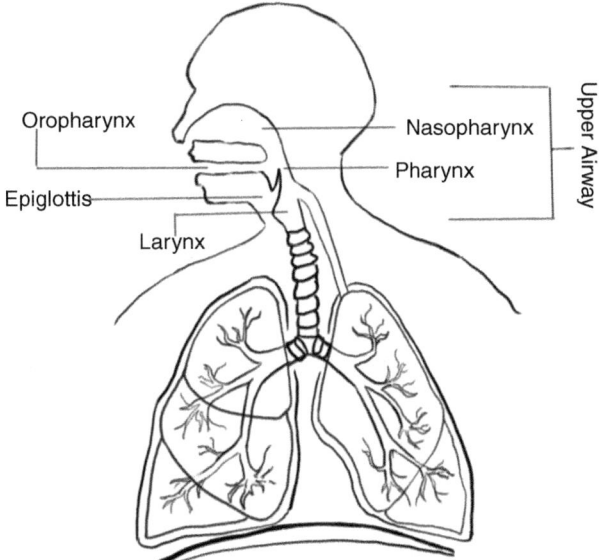

Lower Airway

The *trachea* is the tube through which air travels into the lungs and connects to the bronchi.

The *bronchi* split the air coming from the trachea between the two lungs.

The *bronchioles* branch off of the two bronchi to bring air throughout the lungs.

The *alveoli* are pockets at the end of the bronchioles where the actual diffusion of oxygen into the bloodstream, and vice versa with carbon dioxide, occurs.

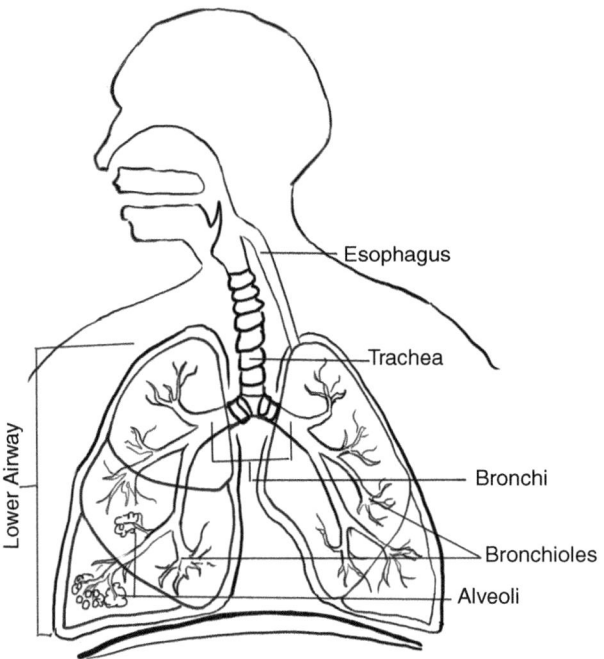

Blood Pressure

Learning Objectives
Upon completing this section, you should be able to

- *understand* biological regulation of blood pressure,
- *identify* hypotension and hypertension,
- *infer* effects of hypotension,
- *communicate* methods of blood pressure assessment.

Blood pressure assessment is one of the most important tools in a healthcare provider's tool kit. This value can assist us in understanding a patient's internal status, stability, and condition. We say that blood pressure is equal to cardiac output minus vascular resistance and is measured in millimeters of mercury (mmHg). An adult's normal resting blood pressure is typically $\frac{120}{80}$ mmHg with the top number called the *systolic* and the bottom number called *diastolic*. The systolic value represents the peak fluid pressure at *systole*, while the diastolic value represents blood pressure through arteries at *diastole*. *Pulse pressure* refers to the difference in the systolic and diastolic blood pressure. For example, a blood pressure of $\frac{136}{54}$ mmHg would equate to a pulse pressure of 82 mmHg. Stroke volume represents the actual volume of blood that is released with each heartbeat. We get our *cardiac output* value by adding stroke volume and pulse pressure.

Systolic Blood Pressure Indicators
- *Normal*: 120 mmHg (±8)
- *Hypotension*: ≤90 mmHg
- *Stage I hypertension:* 130–139 mmHg
- *Stage II hypertension*: ≥140 mmHg
- *Hypertensive crisis*: ≥180 mmHg

The most prevalent blood pressure regulatory mechanism you should be concerned about is the *renin-angiotensin-aldosterone system (RAAS)*, which works to increase overall arterial blood pressure. Before we can tackle RAAS, we first need to understand the relationship between blood pressure and vascular surface area. Imagine you have a coffee stirrer and a milkshake (or bubble tea) straw. The diameters are noticeably different. Which straw would you say is easier to blow through? If you're not sure, try it! You'll notice that intuitively, a larger diameter corresponds with less pressure needed to blow through. This is exactly what happens when we talk about arterial blood pressure! As vessels dilate, BP decreases. This is called *vasodilation*. As vessels constrict, BP increases. This is called *vasoconstriction*. It's important to note that heat stimulus usually causes vasodilation to allow vessels to come closer to the surface of the skin to cool down, while cold stimulus causes vasoconstriction. *Preload* is referred to as the pressure remaining during diastole, while *afterload* refers to the pressure that must be created to allow for blood flow to the aorta.

If you've ever heard of ACE inhibitors for the treatment of high blood pressure, you're already ahead of the game! As previously mentioned, the purpose of RAAS is to increase BP, and it starts with the kidneys. The short and sweet story begins with the production of renin at the juxtaglomerular cells within the kidney. Renin is circulated until it meets with angiotensinogen secreted by the liver. When renin and angiotensinogen meet, angiotensin I is made. When this hormone is met with an enzyme known as *angiotensin converting enzyme (ACE)*, angiotensin II is created, which is our desired product. Angiotensin II is a powerful vasoconstrictor which is the primary resulting mechanism which increases BP in this system.

Critical Skill: *Blood Pressure by Auscultation*
- *Step 1:* Obtain access to the antecubital fossa and palpate for a brachial pulse.
- *Step 2:* Apply the sphygmomanometer cuff superior to the antecubital fossa.
- *Step 3:* Place the stethoscope on the antecubital fossa, and inflate the cuff until the Korotkoff sounds (thumping) are not audible.
- *Step 4:* Begin to deflate slowly, and note the start of the Korotkoff sounds, the systolic blood pressure, and the ending of the sounds, the diastolic blood pressure.
- *Step 5:* Deflate and remove the sphygmomanometer cuff.

Critical Skill: *Blood Pressure by Palpation*
- *Step 1:* Obtain access to the antecubital fossa and palpate for brachial pulse.
- *Step 2:* Apply the sphygmomanometer cuff superior to the antecubital fossa.
- *Step 3:* Palpate for a radial pulse and inflate until it cannot be felt anymore.
- *Step 4:* Begin to deflate slowly, and note the start of when the radial pulse can be felt, the systolic blood pressure. Note that a diastolic blood pressure cannot be measured via palpation.
- *Step 5:* Deflate and remove the sphygmomanometer cuff.

Respiratory Emergencies

Learning Objectives
Upon completing this section, you should be able to

- *understand* the progression of untreated respiratory emergencies,
- *identify* a patient in respiratory distress,
- *infer* causes of respiratory emergencies,
- *communicate* an understanding of the role of compensatory mechanisms.

Respiratory emergencies are a leading cause of death in the United States, and it is true that the majority of lethal respiratory conditions are preventable with immediate lifesaving interventions. Adequate breath relies on the integrated processes of ventilation, oxygenation, and respiration. *Ventilation* is the act of facilitating air movement in and out of the lungs by muscles and other structures. *Oxygenation* is the process of storing available oxygen molecules into hemoglobin in red blood cells. *Respiration* describes the concurrent gas exchange of oxygen and carbon dioxide molecules in both tissues and the alveoli. In a singular breath, the quantity of air that is facilitated in and out of the lungs is called the *tidal volume*, while *residual volume* describes the amount of air that remains after complete exhalation.

Inhalation

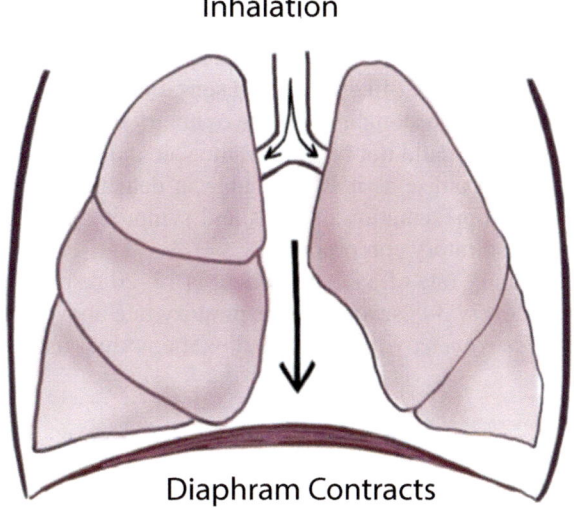

Diaphram Contracts

Exhalation

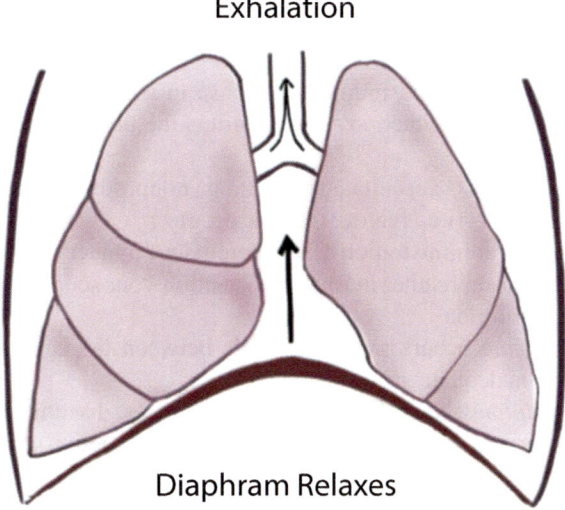

Diaphram Relaxes

When a patient is unable to adequately deliver oxygen to bodily tissues, this is known as *hypoxia*. A common indicator of hypoxia is *cyanosis*, which occurs when the skin turns blue due to poor oxygenation. Cyanosis can either be peripheral or central and is usually associated with late-stage respiratory distress. The presence of *subcutaneous emphysema* is also a reliable indication of hypoxia and occurs when air is trapped in tissues underneath chest and neck skin. When affected skin tissue is palpated, it produces a crackling-like sound and sensation known as *crepitus*.

Hypoxia is also known to accompany a pulse oximetry reading below 94%; however, the use of oximetry should not be used as the sole indicator for the identification of respiratory compromise as it is unreliable in detecting rapid changes in a patient's status. Clinical presentation of signs and symptoms remains as the most reliable indicator of respiratory compromise.

The regular respiratory rate of an adult patient is 12–20 respirations per minute (RPM) or one breath every 3–5 seconds. A respiratory rate above the normal range is considered to be *tachypneic*, while a rate below the normal range is *dyspneic* or *bradypnea*.

Normal Respiratory Rates
- *Adult*: 12–20 RPM
- *Child*: 15–30 RPM
- *Infant*: 25–50 RPM
- *Newborn*: 40–60 RPM (30–40 RPM minutes after delivery)

Asthma is an exaggerated immune response in the lower respiratory tract that induces bronchospasms, which in turn constricts the bronchioles and fills its inner lining with mucus.

Signs and symptoms: auscultated wheezing, nonproductive cough, and associated allergy symptoms (i.e., red eyes, sneezing, etc.)

Treatment: assist administration of a metered dose inhaler (MDI); high-flow oxygen therapy via non-rebreather mask; and, if within your scope, nebulized albuterol and ipratropium bromide

Pulmonary edema occurs when fluid fills between the capillaries and alveoli, which results in inadequate gas exchange.

Signs and symptoms: auscultated crackles, cyanosis, discomfort when breathing supine (orthopnea), productive cough (pink and frothy sputum), and signs of edema in other regions

Treatment: high-flow oxygen via positive pressure ventilation

Pneumonia is a condition secondary to a viral or bacterial infection in the lower airway that causes fluid to fill the alveoli.

Signs and symptoms: auscultated crackles, chest discomfort, fever, general malaise, productive cough associated with bacterial pneumonia, and nonproductive cough associated with viral pneumonia

Treatment: high-flow oxygen therapy

Spontaneous pneumothorax occurs when a lung partially collapses and visceral lining ruptures. This type of pneumothorax is not secondary to traumatic injury and usually occurs in patients with a history of COPD.

Signs and symptoms: decreased auscultated lung sounds over one side, sharp chest discomfort, subcutaneous emphysema, and tracheal deviation

Treatment: oxygen therapy if indicated

Tension pneumothorax occurs when trauma induces a lung to collapse, usually secondary to a sucking chest wound. As with most pneumothoraces, a mediastinal shift in the opposite direction of the sucking chest wound is common.

Signs and symptoms: decreased auscultated lung sounds over one side, sharp chest discomfort, obvious penetrating chest trauma, and tracheal deviation

Treatment: application of a chest seal if indicated and oxygen therapy

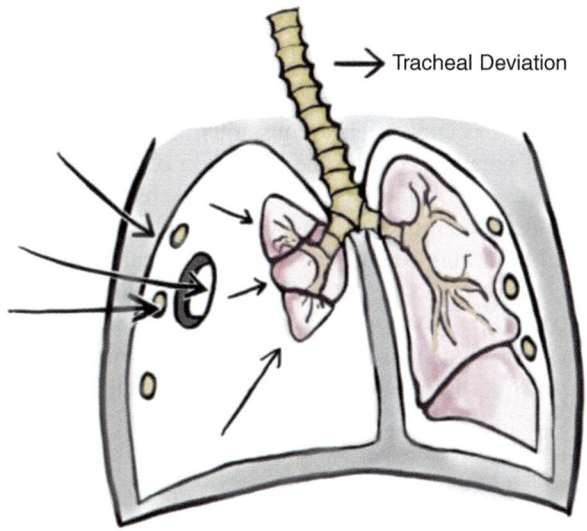

Tracheal Deviation

Tension Pneumothorax

Hyperventilation, usually secondary to anxiety, occurs when a patient exhales faster than they inhale, which results in a rapid reduction of carbon dioxide and thus an unproportionate balance of gases.

Signs and symptoms: altered mental status, numbness and tingling, dizziness, and sometimes seizures in patients with a history of epilepsy

Treatment: oxygen therapy if indicated and emotional support

Pulmonary embolism occurs when a clot, air, fat, or other object obstructs a pulmonary artery.

Signs and symptoms: altered mental status, numbness and tingling, dizziness, and sometimes seizures in patients with a history of epilepsy

Treatment: oxygen therapy if indicated and emotional support

Chronic obstructive pulmonary disease (COPD) is a general term for prolonged airway obstruction and includes emphysema and bronchitis.

Emphysema is characterized by decreased lung elasticity and moderate to severe alveolar damage.

Signs and symptoms: barrel chest and nonproductive cough

Treatment: oxygen therapy if indicated and, if within your scope, nebulized albuterol and ipratropium bromide

Bronchitis is characterized by bronchial inflammation and exorbitant production of mucus.

Signs and symptoms: auscultated wheezing, rales, and cough

Treatment: oxygen therapy if indicated and, if within your scope, nebulized albuterol and ipratropium bromide

Assessment of a patient's breathing relies on rate, rhythm, quality, lung sounds, chest rise and fall, work of effort, and depth.

Respiratory compromise describes any form of respiratory insufficiency and occurs when a patient is unable to adequately and appropriately engage in any aspect of normal respiration:

1. *Respiratory distress* occurs when a conscious patient presents with increased work of effort of breathing due to the activation of homeostatic compensatory mechanisms. *Signs and symptoms*: tachycardia, tachypnea, nasal flaring, pursed lips, head bobbing, stridor or wheezing, and altered mental status.
2. *Respiratory failure* occurs when there is poor oxygenation and/or ventilation to meet the demands of organ systems. There are limited available compensatory mechanisms. *Signs and symptoms*: bradycardia, dyspnea, grunting, delayed capillary refill, cyanosis, hypotension, and damp and clammy skin.
3. *Respiratory arrest* occurs when an unresponsive patient stops breathing but still has a palpable carotid pulse. *Signs and symptoms*: minimal or no air flow, inefficient respiratory effort (inadequate chest rise and fall), and cyanosis.

Respiratory compromise encompasses the events of rapid deterioration of a patient's respiratory status. It is critical that providers initiate appropriate oxygen therapy to prevent worsening of a patient's condition.

Check Your Understanding: *Respiratory Compromise*
You are responding to a 34-year-old male patient with shortness of breath. He has a history of COPD emphysema, type 1 diabetes, and an allergy to penicillin. Upon auscultation, you noticed decreased lung sounds over the left side of this posterior thorax. What condition is this patient most likely experiencing?

Respiratory Treatment and Pharmacology

Learning Objectives
Upon completing this section, you should be able to

- *understand* basic mechanisms of respiratory pharmacology,
- *identify* when oxygen therapy may be indicated,
- *infer* which oxygen delivery device may be appropriate,
- *communicate* when ALS intervention may be needed.

Effective management of a patient's airway and breathing is a major responsibility of the EMS provider that can significantly affect a patient's prognosis. When a patient's airway is conducive to normal ventilatory function, we say their airway is *patent*. Normal respiration should be comfortable and require minimal effort. When the airway is not patent, such as due to the presence of a *foreign body airway obstruction* (*FBAO*), the airway is deemed *compromised*.

Special sounds can indicate if an airway is compromised:

– *Snoring* is indicative of a partial upper airway obstruction, often the tongue. Treatment may be as simple as adjusting the airway via the jaw thrust maneuver or the head-tilt/chin-lift method. If basic airway modifications prove ineffective, consider inserting an oropharyngeal airway.
– *Gurgling* is indicative of fluid in the upper airway, such as secretions. Treatment involves immediate suctioning and the use of a basic airway maneuver or oral adjunct if appropriate.
– *Rhonchi* is a snoring-like sound that can be produced from either the upper or lower airway that is indicative of excessive mucus production.

Basic airway maneuvers:

The *head-tilt/chin-lift* maneuver is an easy option to open a supine patient's airway. This maneuver should not be performed on patients suspected of having cervical spinal injuries, as it could cause further injury.

Critical Skill: *Head-Tilt/Chin-Lift Maneuver*
• *Step 1:* Place one hand on the patient's forehead.
• *Step 2:* Place 2–3 fingers on the other hand under the mandible.
• *Step 2:* Simultaneously push down on the forehead and up on the mandible.

The *jaw thrust* maneuver is traditionally considered for patients who require additional cervical spine precautions.

Critical Skill: *Jaw Thrust Maneuver*
• *Step 1:* Place hands on both sides of the posterior area of the patient's mandible with fingers curled.
• *Step 2:* Push the mandible up and away from the patient's neck.

Critical Skill: *Inserting an OPA*
• *Step 1:* Select the appropriately sized OPA by measuring the distance from the corner of the mouth to the earlobe or to the angle of the jaw and selecting a similarly sized OPA.
• *Step 2:* Open the airway by performing either a jaw thrust or head-tilt/chin-lift maneuver.

- *Step 3:* Visualize the patient's oropharynx by using a cross-finger or scissor technique, and check for any airway obstructions.
- *Step 4*:* Insert the OPA in the direction opposite to the anatomical airway till the tip reaches the hard palate.
- *Step 5:* Rotate the airway 180°, and insert till the end or the airway is resting on or slightly above the patient's lips.
  *The OPA may be placed perpendicular to the anatomical airway and rotated 90° if a tongue depressor is available to move the tongue out of the way.

Critical Skill: *Inserting an NPA*
- *Step 1:* Select the appropriately sized NPA by measuring the distance from the nose to the earlobe and selecting a similarly sized NPA.
- *Step 2:* Lubricate the tip of the NPA.
- *Step 3:* Insert the NPA such that the bevel is toward the nasal septum.
- *Step 4:* Advance the NPA until the flange is just outside the nose.

Positive airway pressure (PAP) ventilation is an essential skill within the BLS scope that is used for patients who cannot breathe on their own. Methods include the following:

- Mouth to mask ventilation
- One or two rescuer bag valve mask (BVM) ventilation
- Continuous positive airway pressure (CPAP) machine ventilation

Critical Skill: *Use of a BVM With One Rescuer*
Step 1: Properly assemble the BVM.
- *Step 2:* Place the mask portion of the BVM on the patient's face with the more narrow area on the nose.
- *Step 3:* Assume an E-C grip in which one's index finger and thumb are around the tubular portion of the mask below the valve and the remaining three fingers are around the patient's mandible.
- *Step 4:* In the E-C position, manually open the airway by pulling the patient's head slightly back.
- *Step 5:* With the free hand, squeeze the bag portion of the BVM such that there is full chest rise and fall 10–12 breaths per minute or one breath every 5–6 seconds unless directed otherwise by medical direction or protocols.
  *Attach BVM to an oxygen source at 15 LPM or higher when available.

You may encounter a patient with a *tracheal stoma*, which is a small tube connected to the trachea which allows a patient to breathe without the use of their upper airway. Ventilation can be provided by covering the stoma hole and providing traditional BVM ventilation. Alternatively, the mask can be removed, and the bag of the BVM can be directly attached to the tube. Ventilation should be provided at a rate of one breath every 5–6 seconds connected to high-flow oxygen at 15 LPM.

Oxygen therapy is the priority treatment for patients experiencing respiratory compromise. In the prehospital setting, the source of oxygen gas (O2) is delivered by a *tank*. The internal O2 capacity relies on the size of the tank at a given pressure, traditionally measured in pounds per square inch (PSI). A full tank is typically around 2000 PSI.

O2 cylinder type	O2 capacity (at ~2000 PSI)
A	113 L
B	165 L
C	255 L
D	425 L
E	680 L

Oxygen therapy can be administered using a variety of oxygen delivery tools:

- A *simple mask* is given at a rate of 5–10 LPM and is rarely used.
- A *nasal cannula* is given at a rate of 2–6 LPM and delivers an O2 concentration of approximately 30%. It is indicated for patients who can ventilate themselves and only require a little amount of oxygen. This device is not sufficient for patients in respiratory compromise.
- A *non-rebreather mask* is given at a rate of 10–15 LPM and delivers an O2 concentration of approximately 90%. It is indicated for patients who can ventilate themselves but require a high concentration of oxygen due to medical or traumatic circumstances.
- A *bag valve mask* is given and delivers an O2 concentration of approximately 90%. It is indicated for patients who cannot ventilate themselves adequately and require the highest concentration of oxygen due to medical or traumatic circumstances such as respiratory arrest.
- A *continuous positive airway pressure* (CPAP) device is indicated in patients with acute pulmonary edema. Check your local protocols to verify if this is within your scope of practice.

Providers should be mindful that not every patient needs oxygen therapy. In fact, the administration of unindicated supplementary oxygen can be very detrimental to some patient populations. Extra precaution should be given to patients with a history of COPD, as only a nasal cannula device is typically indicated. Oxygen toxicity should be prevented in patients experiencing cardiac compromise, as high amounts of oxygen could warrant inappropriate vasoconstriction.

Some patients with respiratory illness, such as asthma, are prescribed *metered dose inhalers* (*MDI*) that are beta agonists. Most EMS providers are allowed to assist in the administration of a patient's MDI if clinically indicated.

Critical Skill: Assist Administration of an MDI
- *Step 1:* Ensure all the "5 Rights of Drug Administration" are met.
- *Step 2:* Place the medication canister into the actuator and remove the end cap.
- *Step 3:* Direct the patient to place the mouthpiece of the MDI in their mouth making a seal with their lips.
- *Step 4:* Have the patient exhale completely, and then push down on the canister, and have the patient then breathe in slowly.
- *Step 5:* Administer oxygen and repeat if dosage is more than one puff.

Patients who are experiencing respiratory compromise and have a prescribed epinephrine auto-injector should attempt to use it. Here are some quick facts about the drug:

- Epinephrine auto-injectors are administered intramuscularly (IM).
- The dosage is 0.3 mg for adult patients and 0.15 mg (half that of an adult) for pediatric patients.
- Auto-injectors are meant to be administered through clothing.
- Expiration date should always be checked prior to administration.
- Immediate transport is always indicated after administration.

Critical Skill: Assist Administration of an Epinephrine Auto-injector
- *Step 1:* Ensure all the "5 Rights of Drug Administration" are met.
- *Step 2:* Have the patient sit down and link hands together, looking in the direction opposite to you.
- *Step 3:* Firmly hold the patient's leg to avoid incomplete administration or breakage of the needle.
- *Step 4:* Remove the safety cap from the epinephrine auto-injector, and hold in line with the largest part of the patient's thigh.
- *Step 5:* Move the auto-injector slightly back and then forcefully forward to inject the epinephrine, and hold for 3 seconds.
- *Step 6:* Remove the auto-injectors straight out, and have the patient gently rub the area for 10 seconds to disperse the medication.

Check Your Understanding: *Oxygen Delivery*
You are responding to an 18-year-old female patient with shortness of breath in a tripod position. She has a history of mild asthma. Which of the following should be your first immediate intervention?

(a) Apply a cervical collar.
(b) Assist the patient with her inhaler.
(c) Ventilate the patient with a BVM, 1 breath every 5–6 seconds.
(d) Apply a non-rebreather mask at 15 LPM.

Cardiac Emergencies

Learning Objectives
Upon completing this section, you should be able to

- *understand* the mechanics of cardiac emergencies and how to treat them,
- *identify* cardiac emergencies from symptomatology,
- *infer* how cardiac emergencies are caused,
- *communicate* when treatment is indicated for each emergency.

Acute myocardial infarction, commonly known as a heart attack, occurs when the heart tissue dies due to a blockage of blood supply. Blockage causing inadequate or no perfusion of blood is called *ischemia*, while the resulting tissue death is an *infarction*. If not treated immediately, an acute myocardial infarction could lead to a cardiac arrest. Infarcted heart muscle cannot return to its original state, even if it repairs itself. So, even if the patient survives the initial heart attack, they are open to many more future cardiac issues.

Symptoms: diaphoresis (sweating), nausea, weakness, syncope, shortness of breath, substernal chest pressure, pain radiating into the left jaw and shoulder, and lower back and abdominal pain

Treatment: 162–325 mg aspirin (acetylsalicylic acid) PO, chewed, and nitroglycerin (as prescribed)

When it comes to symptoms of an acute MI, they differ biologically between males and females, but no symptoms are exclusive to one sex or another. Males usually experience chest pain and pain that radiates into the left jaw and/or shoulder. Females are more likely to experience abdominal and lower back discomfort. Female patients have been known to mistake acute MI symptoms as cramping or gastrointestinal issues.

Angina pectoris refers to chest pain that comes from temporary inadequate perfusion to the heart muscle itself. What makes it differ from an acute MI is that, although both stem from cardiac ischemia (with the exception of vasospastic angina), the blood vessel obstruction is not complete or is temporary. There are three different types of angina:

- *Stable angina* is when the blood vessels are constricted from exercise and in turn become blocked. So, if there is buildup in the vessels, blood may be able to pass when the vessels are large and dilated, but when the available space in the blood vessels becomes smaller due to constriction, the buildup takes up a larger percentage of the space and affects perfusion more. This type of angina can be identified if the chest pain goes away upon cessation of physical activity.
- *Unstable angina* occurs when there is a blockage even when the blood vessels are not constricted. This type of angina is identifiable by the fact that cessation of physical activity does not resolve the pain.
- *Vasospastic angina* is a congenital disorder which causes the blood vessels around the heart to randomly dilate and constrict. Unlike the other two types of angina, this condition is lifestyle dependent. Patients will likely have been diagnosed with this and inform you of it when you take a patient history.

Check Your Understanding: *Angina Pectoris*
You arrive at the scene of a 50-year-old male complaining of chest pain. While taking a patient history, the patient reports that the pain started while he was mowing the lawn but lessened gradually when he sat down to wait for the ambulance. What type of angina does this patient have?

Treatment: 162–325 mg aspirin and nitroglycerin (as prescribed)
Congestive heart failure occurs when the heart valves are too damaged to fully pump blood and fluid starts to back up into the body or the pulmonary veins. It is found in patients who have previously had a myocardial infarction or other condition that has weakened the heart muscle.
    Symptoms: pedal edema (swelling around the feet, legs, and ankles), productive coughing (sometimes with blood in the mucus), shortness of breath, irregular heart rate, tachycardia, and jugular vein distention
    Cardiac tamponade occurs when pressure is put on the heart due to fluid filling the pericardium or the sac that surrounds the heart. The symptomology for a cardiac tamponade is organized in Beck's triad:
    Beck's triad

- Muffled heart sounds
- Jugular vein distention
- Low pulse pressure (<25 mmHg)

Aortic dissection occurs when an aortic aneurysm, a weak spot in the wall of the aorta, ruptures and blood from the aorta causes pressure which separates and tears the layers of the aorta.

Symptoms: severe, sharp chest and back pain; nausea; and mismatched radial pulsed

Acetylsalicylic acid (ASA), or simply aspirin, is a nonsteroidal anti-inflammatory (NSAID) drug that interferes with normal blood platelet functioning and is indicated in acute cardiac compromise. Aspirin should always be chewed if given for this purpose. Contraindications include gastrointestinal bleeding or surgery within the past four months, allergy to aspirin, or physician direction to never take aspirin. Geriatric patients are often advised by their primary care provider to take 81 mg (baby aspirin) daily for preventative measures.

Nitroglycerin is a vasodilator that decreases chest pain by dilating ischemic vessels and is indicated in a suspected acute myocardial infarction for patients who are prescribed it. Dosage varies between 0.3 and 0.6 mg and is administered sublingually. This drug is contraindicated in patients who have taken erectile dysfunction medicine in the past 48 hours or have a low systolic pressure (less than 100 mmHg). Because nitroglycerin is a powerful vasodilator, it can cause a precipitous drop in blood pressure and can be lethal if administered improperly. It is important that you communicate to your patient that one of the risks of administering nitroglycerin after having taken erectile dysfunction is possible death. Always familiarize yourself with local protocols, and contact medical control with any questions or concerns.

Check Your Understanding: *Acute Cardiac Compromise*
You are treating an elderly male patient whom you suspect to be having a heart attack. You administer 325 mg of aspirin and identify that the patient has been prescribed nitroglycerin by his cardiologist. You note the following vital signs: HR: 106 BPM, RR: 14 RPM, BP: 116/p, and O2: 98%. What question might you want to ask your patient before administering nitroglycerin?

Chapter Summary

Section "Airway and Cardiothoracic Anatomy"
- Airway, breathing, and circulation are the crux of good emergency medical care. We say that without a patent airway, we have impaired breathing and, inevitably, impaired circulation.
- Maintenance of ABCs comprises the EMS clinician's most critical priority.

Section "Blood Pressure"
- Blood pressure is a critical diagnostic tool for understanding a patient's internal status, condition, and stability.
- The *renin-angiotensin-aldosterone system* (*RAAS*) plays a role in increasing arterial blood pressure through *vasoconstriction*.

Section "Respiratory Emergencies"

- *Ventilation* is the act of facilitating air movement in and out of the lungs by muscles and other structures. *Oxygenation* is the process of storing available oxygen molecules into hemoglobin in red blood cells. *Respiration* describes the concurrent gas exchange of oxygen and carbon dioxide molecules in both tissues and the alveoli.
- When a patient is unable to adequately deliver oxygen to bodily tissues, this is known as *hypoxia*. A common indicator of hypoxia is *cyanosis*, which occurs when the skin turns blue due to poor oxygenation.

Section "Respiratory Treatment and Pharmacology"

- Effective management of a patient's airway and breathing is a major responsibility of the EMS provider. When a patient's airway is conducive to normal ventilatory function, we say their airway is *patent*. Normal respiration should be comfortable and require minimal effort.
- Oxygen therapy is an immediate priority for patients in respiratory compromise, and many devices exist to deliver low and high concentrations of O2.

Section "Cardiac Emergencies"

- *Acute myocardial infarction*, commonly known as a heart attack, occurs when the heart tissue dies due to a blockage of blood supply. Blockage causing inadequate or no perfusion of blood is called *ischemia*, while the resulting tissue death is an *infarction.*
- If an acute MI is not treated immediately, it could lead to a cardiac arrest.

Practice Questions

1. A patient tells you that "I was running a marathon and my chest started to really hurt, but when I rested, the pain started to fade." What medical issue does this indicate?

    (a) Stable angina
    (b) Unstable angina
    (c) Vasospastic angina
    (d) Myocardial infarction

2. You arrive on scene to a patient with a dull, heavy, chest pain. What medication are you allowed to give them without a prior prescription?

    (a) Nitroglycerin
    (b) Aspirin
    (c) Epinephrine
    (d) Morphine

3. You arrive on scene to a patient who has a gunshot wound to the chest. Upon assessment, you note absent lung sounds on one side and a deviated trachea. What respiratory emergency is the patient most likely suffering from?

   (a) Pulmonary edema
   (b) Asthma
   (c) Punctured lung
   (d) Tension pneumothorax

4. A patient's blood pressure is 87/45 mmHg. Are they…

   (a) Hypotensive
   (b) Normal
   (c) Hypertensive

Chapter 6
Principles of Basic Life Support

Introduction

Experienced paramedics and other advanced providers often say that "good advanced life support arises from the foundation of good basic life support." A strong understanding of BLS principles will serve you well in any medical career.

In this chapter, you will understand the scope of practice and role of a BLS provider. You will learn how to recognize a cardiac arrest, perform high-quality CPR, and use an automated external defibrillator. This chapter will assist you in building your clinical intuition for understanding when life support is indicated and how to deliver it effectively in accordance with the latest resuscitation science.

Cardiac Arrest

Learning Objectives
Upon completing this section, you should be able to

- *understand* the pathophysiology of a cardiac arrest,
- *identify* the signs and symptoms of a patient in cardiac arrest,
- *infer* possible causes of a cardiac arrest,
- *communicate* how to care for a patient in cardiac arrest.

You might often come across newspaper headlines such as "Local woman saves man from a heart attack by doing CPR," but this wording is clinically incorrect. In Chap. 5, you learned that a heart attack is a blockage in an artery that supplies

C. Ventura et al., *The Emergency Medical Responder*,
https://doi.org/10.1007/978-3-030-64396-6_6

oxygenated blood to the heart, easily treated at the BLS level with aspirin. So when do you perform CPR?

Cardiac arrest is a condition in which the heart can no longer sufficiently circulate oxygen-rich blood throughout the body, usually due to an irregular heart rhythm. While ALS providers can assess heart rhythms with an ECG machine, BLS providers only check for a pulse. The key characteristic of a cardiac arrest is the lack of a palpable carotid pulse. There are many different medical and traumatic causes for a cardiac arrest, but treatment at a BLS level is essentially standard: the immediate activation of the chain of survival, the use of an AED, ventilations, and CPR.

Most common causes for cardiac arrest	
Hypovolemia	Trauma
Hypoxia	Tamponade
Hypothermia	Thrombosis
Hypoglycemia	Toxins
Hyper/hypokalemia	Tension pneumothorax
Hydrogen ion excess	

Sudden cardiac arrest is cardiac arrest which has no preexisting conditions. This usually occurs when an outside event disrupts the heart rhythm, like being hit in the chest, but sometimes, the cause is unknown. Sudden cardiac arrest is equally likely to occur in people young and old, no matter their health condition.

> **Check Your Understanding: Cardiac Arrest Causes**
> At a school softball game, a child gets hit in the chest with the ball. He/she then collapses to the ground. You run up to the child, and he/she appears to be unresponsive. You find that he/she is not breathing and does not have a pulse. What condition is the patient most likely experiencing? What is the most likely cause of the condition?

Primary Assessment

> **Learning Objectives**
> Upon completing this section, you should be able to
>
> - *understand* how to assess for a pulse and breathing,
> - *identify* if a person is unconscious or unresponsive,
> - *infer* what line of treatment is appropriate for the patient,
> - *communicate* to others when to activate the chain or survival.

In order to be able to properly care for a patient, you must first diagnose the issue that requires treatment. In this section, we will cover the BLS primary assessment, the diagnostic process used by providers at a BLS level. In the BLS primary assessment, we are trying to answer two main questions: whether the patient is in cardiac arrest and whether they are apneic. We can quickly check for these two conditions while following the prescribed steps to determine what actions should be performed and in what order.

To start off our algorithm, we will begin by determining the mental status of our patient. Specifically, we will determine whether our patient is truly unresponsive or merely unconscious. The state of being *unconscious* is very loosely defined, stating only that the patient is not currently awake and alert. On the other hand, an *unresponsive* patient is one who is unable to be roused by either verbal or painful stimuli. Examples of situations in which a person is considered unresponsive include patients in cardiac and respiratory arrest as well as those who are in a coma or under general anesthesia.

As mentioned previously, we will attempt to arouse our patient using both verbal and painful stimuli. In order to assess verbal stimuli, ask the patient in a loud voice whether they are okay. Repeat the question several times. If they fail to respond, move on to painful stimuli. There are several options for painful stimuli, all of which are designed to cause strong sensations of pain without injuring the patients. The first option is three firm blows to the upper chest. This is the simplest method and the one most often taught in BLS classes for lay and professional rescuers. Two alternative methods of assessing response to painful stimuli are known as the sternal rub and the trapezius pinch. A *sternal rub* is a maneuver in which one takes two knuckles and forcefully applies pressure to the patient's sternum while rubbing up and down. This method is commonly used by EMS and healthcare professionals. A *trapezius pinch* is a maneuver in which one uses their index finger and thumb to apply firm pressure to the trapezius muscle along the backside of the shoulder. When looking for a response to these stimuli, keep in mind that the patient may not show responsiveness by completely awakening, but may instead show a response through either a change in facial expression and position or a flinch or withdrawal from the stimuli. If the patient is found to not be unresponsive, we can continue with either the medical or trauma assessment. If the patient is unresponsive, we continue the BLS primary assessment.

Now that we have determined that our patient is unresponsive, we want to activate the chain of survival. The *chain of survival* is a set of actions designed to get the patient proper care as quickly as possible, in order to give the patient the highest likelihood of survival. The chain of survival includes such things as calling EMS (if not already present), BLS and ALS treatment, definitive in-hospital care, and post-cardiac arrest care.

At this point in the algorithm, we are unsure whether the patient is in cardiac or respiratory arrest. However, because the patient is unresponsive, we know that there is a major medical issue. Knowing this, we want to activate the chain of survival. This may change depending on whether you are currently on or off duty. If you are not on shift, tell a bystander to call 911, and tell a different bystander to get an AED. When doing this, you want to be very specific in who you are directing to perform which actions. Do this by pointing at the person you are talking to and using specific identifiers such as "you, the woman in red shirt, call 911" and "you in the jersey, go get an AED." If the person does not immediately do so, move on to another person.

This process is designed to avoid the bystander effect, where everyone in a group assumes another person will act. Calling out to a specific person subverts this.

If you are on shift, your response should obviously be different. Remember that **you** are 911, and take action accordingly. First, determine that your patient is unresponsive, and activate the chain of survival. Get the AED from your equipment, and request that an ALS unit be dispatched to assist in the care of the patient. If you are working in an in-hospital setting, the chain of survival can simply be activated by pushing the blue button, which will call a code blue, informing the hospital of an unresponsive patient. The appropriate providers will arrive to care for the patient.

Once the chain of survival has been activated, we want to determine if the patient is in cardiac arrest or respiratory arrest so that we can provide appropriate treatment. We can assess the patient using a process called "look, listen, and feel." We want to look for chest rise and fall. When assessing breathing, we also want to place our ear close to the patient's mouth to both listen and feel for breathing. During this assessment, you may see *agonal respirations*, which is random gasping caused by a response in the central nervous system. This is not considered to be breathing. It is important that we also assess cardiac function, which can be done by feeling for a pulse. When assessing for a pulse, we check the carotid artery. If there is a lack of pulse at the carotid artery, it can be assumed that it is also not present at other locations. Checking for a pulse is done by placing the index and middle fingers on the neck beside the trachea with light pressure. In order to minimize the amount of time before treatment is initiated, it is important that you simultaneously check for breathing and a pulse. Assess for 5–10 seconds. This time window will identify breathing or pulse in the case of severe dyspnea or bradycardia without delaying care more than necessary. If there is a pulse and breathing, move on to completing a medical or trauma assessment. Alternatively, if the patient is not breathing but has a pulse, move to treating the patient according to the apneic patient algorithm. Finally, if both pulse and breathing are not present, our patient is in cardiac arrest, and we will continue with the appropriate treatment.

Check Your Understanding: BLS Primary Assessment
You are called to an unconscious male who was found unconscious under a bridge. After ensuring the scene is safe and proper personal protective equipment is donned, you check for response to verbal and painful stimuli and conclude that the patient is unresponsive. What would be the next appropriate action to be performed for this patient?

(a) Begin chest compressions.
(b) Have your partner request ALS and bring the AED.
(c) Check for a pulse or breathing.
(d) Perform a detailed neurological assessment.

High-Quality CPR

Learning Objectives
Upon completing this section, you should be able to

- *understand* how fast and deep to perform compressions,
- *identify* where to perform compressions,
- *infer* if the patient is reviving sufficient circulation,
- *communicate* to others if the quality of compressions is adequate.

When a patient is in cardiac arrest, management of the condition revolves around chest compressions. *Chest compressions* are manual external contractions of a patient's heart, applied through forceful thrusts to the center of the sternum against a flat hard surface. From a physiological standpoint, we are essentially pumping the patient's heart for them by squeezing it between the sternum and a hard surface. When the heart is compressed, the blood is forced out and circulates through the body. This gives the patient more time before major damage occurs, allowing for more definitive treatment to be administered. Though CPR does circulate some blood, it is no substitute for a true heart rhythm and will not sustain a patient indefinitely. This is why additional treatment and the chain of survival are important.

When you are performing chest compressions, you want to be kneeling beside the patient. If your patient is on a stretcher, you want to be at a height where your waistline is slightly above the height of the patient. When preparing for chest compressions, hand placement is key. Begin by taking your dominant hand and placing your nondominant hand on top of it. Interlace the fingers of your nondominant hand while keeping the fingers of your dominant hand fully extended. Place the heel of your bottom hand on the lower third of the sternum or in between the nipple line and the xiphoid process. Ensure that your arms are fully extended and that your back is straight.

Compressions should be performed between 100 and 120 beats per minute. *Staying Alive* by the Bee Gees, with a tempo of 100 BPM, is the song most commonly taught to BLS providers as an example of the proper rhythm. Compressions at this speed balance circulating blood and giving the heart time to refill between compressions. It is important to note that ribs may be broken in this process, but it doesn't indicate that you should cease chest compressions. The ratio of compressions to ventilations is 30:2, meaning that after 30 compressions, you should give two ventilations through methods such as a bag valve mask or pocket mask. It is important that you do not pause compressions for more than 10 seconds. If there is an issue with ventilations which takes more than those 10 seconds, continue with compressions. If there is not an available method for ventilation, you can instead do continuous compressions. The last set of important numbers in chest compressions is how deep each compression should be. Each compression should be 2–2.4 inches deep for the adult patient. The proper depth can be estimated at about 1/3 the depth of the entire patient. When performing compressions, it is also very important that you allow for full chest recoil to allow the heart to refill with blood. As you will learn quickly, chest compressions are very tiring. It is important to know your limits and switch with your partner to take a break if you cannot perform proper chest compressions. Similarly, inform your partner if he or she is not properly performing chest compressions due to fatigue or any other reasons (including lack of knowledge).

As technology improves, there have been innovations in machines which can perform chest compressions. These machines allow the healthcare provider to give other lifesaving interventions. At this time, there are two main types of automated chest compression devices, piston devices and vest devices. A *piston* device is one in which there is an apparatus attached to a hard surface under the patient's chest. The device's mechanical piston will be placed on the patient's sternum and move up and down repeatedly, compressing the patient's chest between the piston and the hard surface. A vest device is very similar, but instead of using a piston, there is a band which contracts around the entire chest of the patient. It is important that you become familiar with how your specific model functions.

Check Your Understanding: BLS Primary Assessment
When providing chest compressions, what combination of rate, ratio, and depth should be performed for the adult patient?

(a) 100–120 BPM, 30:2, 1–2 in
(b) 150–200 BPM, 15:2, 2–2.4 in
(c) 100–120 BPM, 30:2, 2–2.4 in
(d) 50–100 BPM, 10:2, 3–4 in

AED Use

Learning Objectives
Upon completing this section, you should be able to

- *understand* how and when to use an AED,
- *identify* where the AED pads should be placed,
- *infer* when a shock is and is not indicated,
- *communicate* when to clear contact with the patients.

As mentioned previously, one of the possible causes for cardiac arrest is a deadly rhythm known as *ventricular fibrillation*. This is a rhythm where the heart does not have a coordinated electrical pulse. Instead, the random firing of each of the myocytes causes a quivering motion of the ventricles. This rhythm can often occur in people with no preexisting conditions. Thankfully, this is the one rhythm which can receive more treatment than mere management via chest compressions and ventilation.

When a patient is in this rhythm, we can provide what is known as a defibrillation. *Defibrillation* is the administration of a single controlled electrical shock to the heart, "resetting" the heart and introducing an organized cardiac rhythm. One machine that can be used is a manual defibrillator, which allows the provider to determine when a shock is to be administered and how strong of a shock to give based on the analysis of the patient's current cardiac rhythm, often seen on an attached monitor. Unfortunately, you are unable to use one of these devices, as ECG interpretation is an ALS skill. Instead, we can use an AED or *automated external defibrillator*, which is an automated device that identifies ventricular fibrillation and administers the appropriate shock voltage. It is important that, once you determine that your patient is in cardiac arrest, you make use of an AED as soon as possible, even before compressions if possible.

Even though the AED is automated, there are a set of actions you must perform as a provider. The first and most important step is to immediately press the "on" button of the AED. This is important not only because it allows the AED to shock the patient but also because most if not all modern models will provide the rescuer with verbal instructions. When in doubt, follow the AED instructions in the order that they are given. Once the AED is turned on, you will be directed to attach the adhesive pads to both the upper right side of the chest and the lower left side below the rib cage. The pads must be applied to bare skin, and so all clothing on the upper torso must be removed. Each of the pads will have a diagram on them, and it is important to match the diagram to the location on the patient. Once the pads are properly applied to the patient's chest, you can connect the pads to the AED itself. It is important to do these actions in this order, since, once the pads are plugged into the AED, it will begin to analyze electrical activity, and it has no way of knowing whether the pads are attached to the patient. While the AED states that it is analyzing, do not touch the patient. Once the patient has been analyzed by the AED, it will determine whether a shock is indicated. If no shock is indicated, then continue CPR. If a shock is indicated, the AED will begin to charge. You should continue compressions during the charging process, but once the shock is ready to be delivered, you must again cease touching the patient. This is the origin of the "Clear!" often heard in medical dramas; it tells all providers to stop touching the patient. After saying "Clear!" and confirming that no one is touching the patient, press the shock button. Once the shock has been delivered, continue CPR. It is important that you leave the AED pads attached, even if the patient regains consciousness, and allow the AED to reassess every 2 minutes.

Check Your Understanding: AED Use
You are performing compressions on a 40-year-old man who is in cardiac arrest. When an AED arrives at the scene, what is the first action that should be performed?

(a) Apply the pads to the patient.
(b) Administer a defibrillator shock.
(c) Plug in the pad connectors.
(d) Turn on the AED.

Special Considerations

Learning Objectives
Upon completing this section, you should be able to

- *understand* why there may be changes in appropriate treatment,
- *identify* patients which may require special considerations,
- *infer* how treatment should change in different situations,
- *communicate* to team members these changes in procedure.

In any area of medicine, there can be situations in which the standard treatment plan must be altered. For the most part, compressions are standard on every adult patient. However, AED use requires several considerations.

The first and most easily managed complication of AED use is a transdermal patch in the area where a pad needs to be applied. In this situation, remove the patch with a gloved hand, and quickly wipe down the area with an alcohol wipe. Another situation which is quite common among patients is an especially hairy chest. It is possible that the pads will not adhere correctly due to the excess hair. In this situation, you have two main options. The first option is to use the razor which is usually included in the AED kit to shave the area where the pads are to be placed. Alternatively, if the kit does not include a razor but does include an extra set of pads, they can first be applied and then removed to remove the hair before using the second set of new pads to deliver any appropriate shocks. It is important to do this because if the pads are not properly applied, then electrical burns may occur. The third common complication involves patients who have subdermal cardiac implants, such as cardiac pacemakers or internal defibrillators. In these cases, place the pads 2 inches above or below the subdermal device. Lastly, it is important to know whether the patient is in or has recently been in water. Water conducts electrical currents, so it is important that the patient is removed from the water and has their chest quickly dried before the AED pads are applied.

Check Your Understanding: BLS Special Considerations
You find that your pregnant patient is in cardiac arrest. What would be an appropriate change in your treatment plan to account for this special circumstance?

(a) Manually move the uterus to toward the left of the abdomen.
(b) Place the patient in a left lateral recumbent position.
(c) Place AED pads on the front of the sternum and the back or the patient.
(d) Do not provide chest compressions and instead transport immediately.

Airway Obstructions

Learning Objectives
Upon completing this section, you should be able to

- *understand* what the signs of airway obstruction are,
- *identify* if an airway obstruction is complete or incomplete,
- *infer* what treatment is appropriate for the type of airway obstruction,
- *communicate* to the patient to determine if they are choking.

You will often encounter patients who are choking. In medical terms, this is referred to as a "foreign object airway obstruction." A *foreign body airway obstruction* is defined as when an object from the environment lodges itself in the trachea of the patient, impeding proper passage of air both to and from the lungs.

As with cardiac arrest cases, we must determine what condition our patient is experiencing before we can provide proper treatment. A patient who believes they have an airway obstruction will almost always perform the universal sign for choking: the placement of their hands around their throat. In this case, we must determine if there is a complete or partial airway obstruction. In a conscious patient, determine whether they can talk or make any sounds. If the patient is able to cough or make sounds, then a partial airway obstruction is indicated, and you should encourage the patient to continue to cough and attempt to dislodge the object on their own. If there is a complete airway obstruction, intervention is necessary. In most adult patients, we will perform what is known as an abdominal thrust. An *abdominal thrust* is a maneuver in which a forceful blow is applied to the abdomen to expel a foreign body object. This is done by standing behind the patient and wrapping your arms around their abdomen. You will place your dominant hand in a fist with your thumb directed toward the patient and wrap your nondominant hand on the opposite side away from the patient. In this position, you will place your hands above the umbilicus (belly button) and provide a quick forceful movement, inward and upward into the patient's abdomen. Continue performing the maneuver until the foreign body is expelled. In the case of pregnant women, we do not want to harm the fetus, and thus, we will instead perform a chest thrust, which is essentially an abdominal thrust but applied to the center of the sternum. This method can also be used for obese patients.

There are also slight alterations for younger patients. When dealing with pediatric patients, you should still use the abdominal thrust, but you may have to kneel to a more appropriate height. When treating infants, do not perform the abdominal thrust. In caring for these patients, we will instead use back blows and chest compressions. Back blows can be done by placing the infant facing down on your leg while still supporting the head and neck and then applying a forceful blow with the heel of the hand in between the scapula. Chest compressions can be done by holding the patient with one arm, again supporting the head and neck, and then using two fingers applying a quick pressure to the sternum of the infant. Alternate five back blows and five chest compressions until the foreign body is dislodged.

If a patient with a foreign body airway obstruction falls unconscious at any time, perform a head-tilt/chin-lift, and using the scissor technique, manually open the patient's airway. If you can see the obstruction, remove it using a finger sweep, moving your finger under the object and pulling it out. Be sure not to perform a blind finger sweep, as this can cause the object to become lodged deeper into the airway. If an unconscious patient has a foreign body airway obstruction, the treatment is the same for all patients: provide chest compressions as you would in cardiac arrest. You will perform chest compressions until the foreign object is expelled or till ALS services are available. In both conscious and unconscious patients, it is important that they are transported to a hospital so they can be assessed for any other damages.

Check Your Understanding: Foreign Body Airway Obstructions
You are at a family reunion and your brother begins to choke on a piece of his food. He places his hand around his neck, and you hear him coughing. Your mother says that he is choking and then you should provide an abdominal thrust. What would the correct treatment be for this patient?

(a) Provide chest compression.
(b) Provide abdominal thrusts.
(c) Provide back blows.
(d) Encourage continued coughing.

Chapter Summary

Section "Cardiac Arrest"
- *Cardiac arrest* is a condition in which the heart can no longer sufficiently circulate blood throughout the rest of the body, usually due to an irregular heart rhythm, and *sudden cardiac arrest* is cardiac arrest which has no preexisting conditions.
- The most common causes of cardiac arrest can be remembered by the mnemonic "Hs and Ts."

Section "Primary Assessment"
- The state of being *unconscious* is quite broad and is a state in which a patient is not actively aware of any outside stimuli which may occur, and *unresponsiveness* is when one is unable to be roused by either verbal or painful stimuli. Simply put, they cannot be woken up or are stuck in an unconscious state.
- The *chain of survival* is a set of actions that allow for the patient to get the proper care as quickly as possible to give the patient the highest likelihood of survival and should be initiated as soon as possible.
- To determine treatment, the rescuer must assess for a pulse and breathing for 5–10 seconds.

Section "High-Quality CPR"
- *Chest compressions* are the manual external contraction of a patient's heart done by forceful movements of the center of the sternum toward a flat hard surface.
- Chest compression should be done at 100–120 bpm at a depth of 2–2.4 in for adult patients and should be used at a ratio of 30 compressions to two ventilation if possible.

Section "AED Use"
- *Ventricular fibrillation* is a rhythm in which the heart does not have a coordinated electrical pulse but instead a random firing of each of the myocytes causing an overall quivering motion.
- *Defibrillation* is the administration of a single controlled electrical shock provided along through the heart which allows for a restoration of an organized cardiac rhythm, and at the BLS level, an *automated external defibrillator* is an automated device which can identify if the patient is in ventricular fibrillation and administer the appropriate shock voltage.

Section "Special Considerations"
- If a patient has something that is in the area where the AED pads are to be applied, remove it if possible, and clean the area, and if not, move the pad slightly above or below it.
- If the patient is wet, it is important to dry the patient before the use of an AED.
- If the patient is pregnant, displace the fetus to the left side of the abdomen.

Section "Airway Obstructions"
- A *foreign body airway obstruction* is when an object from the environment lodes itself in the trachea of the patient impeding proper passage of air both to and from the lungs.
- An *abdominal thrust* is a maneuver in which a forceful blow is applied to the abdomen to expel a foreign body object. This is done by standing behind the patient but slightly to either side and wrapping your arms around their abdomen.

Practice Questions
1. What special considerations do you need to take for a wet patient when using an AED?

   (a) Make sure to dry the chest before placing the AED pads.
   (b) Lay the patient on a towel before administering a shock.
   (c) Keep their wet clothing on the chest while using the AED.

2. What is the rate of compressions to breaths for a single provider treating a pediatric patient?

   (a) 30–2
   (b) 15–2
   (c) Nonstop compressions
   (d) 30–4

3. What is the rule about the depth of compressions in pediatric patients?

  (a) One-third the depth of the chest
  (b) Two-thirds the depth of the chest
  (c) Half the depth of the chest
  (d) 2–2.4 inches, no matter the size of the patient

4. If your patient is coughing and wheezing due to something lodged in their throat, what kind of airway obstruction do they have?

  (a) Partial airway obstruction.
  (b) Complete airway obstruction.
  (c) Their airway is patented.

Chapter 7
Other Common Medical Emergencies

Introduction

We have previously discussed some medical emergencies that involve the cardiac and respiratory systems, but those are just the tip of the iceberg for pathologies that can occur within the body. Any organ system can manifest problems and cause a medical emergency, and there are many emergencies that affect multiple organ systems. In this chapter, we will go over common medical emergencies that you will experience outside of the two previously discussed categories. These illnesses will vary greatly, covering everything from diabetes, to shock, to heat emergencies.

Endocrine Emergencies

Learning Objectives
Upon completing this section, you should be able to

- *understand* the function of the endocrine system,
- *identify* different endocrinological emergencies,
- *infer* whether the patient is hypoglycemic or hyperglycemic from symptomatology,
- *communicate* with the patient to determine a history of diabetes.

The endocrine system regulates the production of hormones within the body. These hormones act as messengers, each hormone giving a different instruction to the system it affects. In this way, the endocrine system secretes hormones that affect

C. Ventura et al., *The Emergency Medical Responder*, https://doi.org/10.1007/978-3-030-64396-6_7

mood, sleep, metabolism, and more. However, within emergency medicine, the one endocrine process that we are concerned with is glucose metabolism.

Glucose, or sugar, is essential for the body to function and, therefore, needs to be regulated carefully within the body. In order to do this, the pancreas secretes insulin and glucagon. *Insulin* is a hormone that allows glucose to be absorbed into each cell and removes it from the bloodstream. Glucagon is a hormone that can be thought to unlock stored glucose in muscles. The most important point to understand about this process is that the amount of insulin produced and the amount of glucose in the blood are inversely proportional. So if there is a lot of insulin, the blood sugar levels will be low, and if there is no production of insulin, blood sugar levels will be low. The normal and safe blood sugar level is between 80 and 120 mg/dL. This becomes especially important when talking about diabetes, an illness that affects this process.

Diabetes mellitus is a condition where there is a disruption in absorption of glucose into cells. There are two types of diabetes mellitus, and each represents a different way that this disruption is caused:

- Type 1 diabetes, which was previously known as childhood diabetes, is an autoimmune disease where the patient has trouble producing insulin. It was known as childhood diabetes because, unlike the second type of diabetes, the onset of this disease usually occurs in early childhood, although it can present later in life, and it was not caused by lifestyle. Patients take insulin to replace the insulin that their bodies cannot produce and to allow glucose to enter their cells.

Symptoms (new onset): fatigue, polyuria (excessive urination), weight loss, and excessive thirst

- Type 2 diabetes is mostly caused by lifestyle and diet. Excessive consumption of glucose over a long period of time makes the cells resistant to insulin. Unlike type 1, this type of diabetes can be controlled by multiple ways, whether that is through diet or medication.

Diabetic Complications
Hyperglycemia is a condition where the blood sugar level is dangerously high. This is a condition that has a gradual onset, as the glucose level in the blood builds up over time. The general symptoms are warm and dry skin, polydipsia (excessive thirst), increased heart rate, polyuria, polyphagia (excessive hunger), and altered mental status. These general symptoms can occur in both patients with type 1 and type 2 diabetes; however, as the hyperglycemia becomes more severe, more specific illnesses occur:

- *Diabetic ketoacidosis* occurs in patients with type 1 diabetes with severe hyperglycemia. This can occur if the patient has missed multiple insulin shots or their insulin intake is rendered insufficient due to another illness. If untreated, this illness can be fatal, but the onset and progression of the illness take hours.

Symptoms: fruity breath (their breath will have a fruit smell), altered mental status, Kussmaul respirations (fast and deep respirations), nausea and vomiting, and loss of consciousness

Hypoglycemia is a condition where the blood sugar level is dangerously low. This, unlike hyperglycemia, is rapid onset and normally caused by an intake of insulin when the patient has not eaten or taken in enough glucose. This condition can also be found in people who are malnourished without diabetes; however, it is usually to a much lesser extent and is much more rare. Untreated, this condition is fatal.

Symptoms: pale and moist skin, shallow and fast respirations, diaphoresis, tachycardia, altered mental status (many times combative behavior presents), dizziness, seizure, loss of consciousness, and coma

Treatment: oral glucose between cheek and gum

Critical Skill: *Administering Oral Glucose*
1. Verify that oral glucose is indicated in this patient. Consider the patient's history, last oral intake, and blood glucose level if possible.
2. Verify that all five Rs are present.
3. Verify the absence of all contraindications, such as the inability to follow commands, lack of hand strength, or any other indicator of an inadequate gag reflex.
4. If not contraindicated, allow the patient to self-administer the medication. If the glucose comes in gel form, assure the gel is thoroughly spread within the inner cheeks and around the gums before having the patient swallow the remaining gel in the tube. If the glucose comes in tablet form, have the patient chew it. If no commercial form of glucose is available, fruit juice or candy containing a dosage of 15 g of glucose is acceptable.

Fun fact: The State of Vermont includes 15 mL of pure Vermont maple syrup as its official EMS protocol for the treatment of hypoglycemia!

Tip: Remembering the difference between hypoglycemia and hyperglycemia can be tricky, but this rhyme can help:

"Cold and clammy, need some candy. Warm and dry, sugar's high."

Check Your Understanding: *Diabetic Complications*
You arrive at the scene of a 30-year-old male who has had 911 called for him by a bystander reporting erratic behavior. The patient is pale and diaphoretic, and despite not being able to gather a patient history, you notice insulin in the patient's bag. How should you treat this patient?

Environmental Emergencies

Learning Objectives
Upon completing this section, you should be able to

* *understand* the mechanics of heat transfer,
* *identify* temperature-related illnesses from symptomatology,
* *infer* the patient's risk level from observing the environment,
* *communicate* how the patient's body heat should be maintained.

In order to survive and to work efficiently, the body has to maintain a state of homeostasis and has many different internal processes meant to maintain a stable internal environment. One of the most important regulatory processes is the body's ability to regulate temperature. The body requires a very specific temperature to function properly, so when the temperature begins to fluctuate, the body starts to suffer. The environment can affect the temperature of the body through four different processes, convection, conduction, radiation, and evaporation. *Convection* is when heat is transferred to the body through exposure to moving air. *Conduction* is when heat is transferred through direct touch. *Radiation* is when energy, such as heat from the sun or heat from the body, transfers heat. *Evaporation* is when a liquid becomes a gas through an absorption of heat from the surroundings, cooling them. When treating emergencies due to temperature, each of these four processes must be monitored and regulated to help reestablish a stable body temperature.

Heat Emergencies
Heat exhaustion occurs when a heated environment stresses and tires the patient and the body starts to become fatigued. This mostly comes from doing physical or stressful activity in a high-temperature environment; however, pure exposure can cause heat exhaustion as well.

    Symptoms: nausea, vomiting, lightheadedness, general weakness, muscle cramps, thirst, and cool and clammy skin

    Treatment: remove from heat, lie flat, and remove excess cloths

    Heat stroke occurs when the body becomes so overwhelmed by heat that the mechanisms used to maintain body temperature fail. The body has to maintain temperature to function properly, especially the nervous system, so left untreated, heat stroke can be fatal.

    Symptoms: elevated body temperature (above 104 degrees Fahrenheit), may not be sweating, altered mental status, and confusion

    Treatment: immediate transport, lie flat, active cooling, and remove excess clothes

Cold Emergencies
Hypothermia occurs when the body is cooling more than it can produce heat and the body temperature drops to a dangerously low level. It is considered hypothermia

when the body's core temperature drops below 95 degrees Fahrenheit. Symptoms from hypothermia worsen as the temperature falls, and that worsening is categorized into three stages:

– Mild hypothermia is when the core temperature is between 95 and 93 degrees.

Symptoms: shivering and increased respiratory rate
Treatment: remove patient from the cold, remove wet clothing, and cover with emergency blankets

– Moderate hypothermia occurs when the core temperature is between 92 and 86 degrees.

Symptoms: fatigue, confusion, altered mental status, muscle stiffness, lowered respiration rate, lowered heart rate, and feeling of impending doom
Treatment: remove patient from the cold; remove wet clothing; cover with heated blankets; place hot packs at the armpits, neck, and groin; and prevent further heat loss

– Severe hypothermia occurs when the core temperature is less than 86 degrees.

Symptoms: unresponsive, slow and weak heart rate, slow respiration rate, and coma (can progress to cardiac arrest but never assume a cold patient without a palpable distal pulse is dead)
Treatment: if no palpable pulse, begin resuscitation, and rewarming cannot be accomplished in-field but will be done in the hospital; prevent further heat loss

Frostnip is a skin condition where the surface of the skin freezes due to overexposure to the cold. This is most common in places far away from the core that are commonly exposed to air, such as the fingers, ears, and nose. The affected skin will be cold, pale, and numb. Capillary refill will be delayed or absent.

Frostbite is a condition where multiple layers of tissue become frozen, damaging that tissue permanently. Unlike in frostnip, the frozen area will be hard and swollen. The depth of damage caused by frostbite varies due to location and amount of exposure, and symptoms may vary slightly depending on the depth of injury. Frostbite that doesn't pass the layers of the skin may feel thick, but not solid like deeper frostbite.

Abdominal Emergencies

Learning Objectives
Upon completing this section, you should be able to

- *understand* common types of abdominal emergencies,
- *identify* major abdominal organs,
- *infer* possible pathology from clinical presentation,
- *communicate* findings to the receiving facility.

Abdominal emergencies can be some of the most difficult for the EMS provider, as not many assessment methods and treatments are available in the prehospital clinician's toolkit. In fact, generalized abdominal pain is often difficult to diagnose in the emergency room, often requiring a combination of imaging, focused palpation, lab values, and sometimes an ultrasound. The main priority of the prehospital provider for abdominal emergencies includes monitoring the patient's ABCs and providing emotional support.

It is important for you to remember which organ systems lay beneath the abdominal wall so you can get a better understanding of the origin of the emergency:

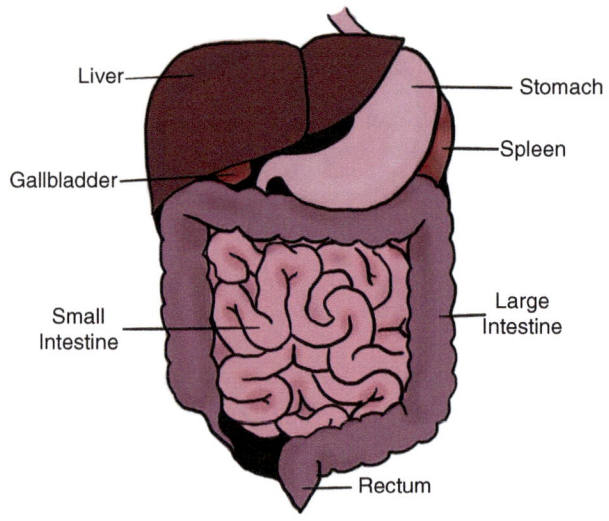

For documentation and reporting purposes, we assign the abdominal region into four quadrants:

- Right upper quadrant (RUQ)
- Left upper quadrant (LUQ)
- Right lower quadrant (RLQ)
- Left lower quadrant (LLQ)

Remember, as with all anatomical terms, that we are referencing the patient's own left and right side. Also, if we describe pain near the belly button, we report this as pain near the *umbilicus*. Every effort to accurately communicate clearly and concisely to receiving medical personnel should be made.

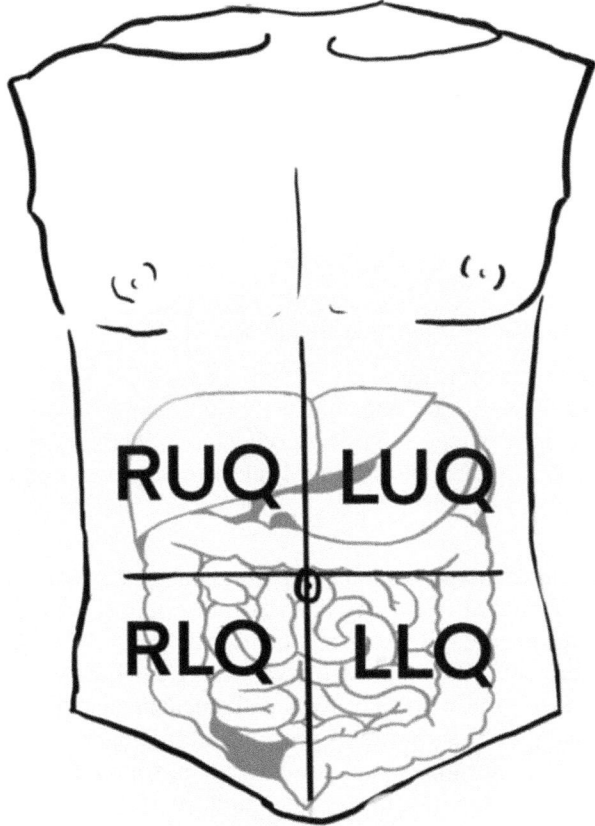

The assessment of the abdomen involves palpation of all four quadrants and auscultating bowel sounds. If the patient complains of pain in a specific region, there is no need to palpate it—note it and move on. Palpation should involve a firm but rolled motion, feeling each quadrant in a clockwise fashion. You should document if you notice any distention or rigidity, which could indicate internal trauma or hemorrhaging. If the patient reflexes to guard a quadrant from your palpation, this is known as *guarding* and is a sign of severe discomfort. You should also note if the patient grimaces when palpation is performed.

When listening for bowel sounds, document if the "rumbling" is absent, hypoactive, or hyperactive. It may take at least 15 seconds to start hearing bowel sounds. Any abnormalities should be reported to the receiving medical team.

Patients with acute abdominal pain always come with a potential for shock. Monitor your patient closely, and reassess vital signs regularly for hypotension or hypoxia. Low-concentration oxygen therapy may be therapeutic for some patients, especially those who are anxious. Provide emotional support by talking to them if the patient is willing, to distract from the pain, and provide a warm blanket if desired. Note that pain over the right lower quadrant to the umbilicus known as "McBurney's point" may be indicative of acute appendicitis.

Poisons and Toxins

Learning Objectives
Upon completing this section, you should be able to

- *understand* what defines a poison,
- *identify* the way a poison enters the body from symptomatology,
- *infer* the identity of a poison by observing the patient's surroundings,
- *communicate* with the poison control center to identify a poison.

Poisons are any substances which chemically damage the body or bodily functions. This is not limited to the big name, deadly poisons like arsenic or cyanide, but includes everyday objects and chemicals that your patients may have come into contact with. Poison is also a very large category for many different types of substances with different effects and mechanisms. One subcategory of poisons is toxins. A *toxin* is an organic poison which damages cells. Recognizing if a poisoning has occurred requires knowledge on some of the different types of poisons and understanding how your patient may have come into contact with said poison. However, on the EMS level, our knowledge on the vast number of poisons is limited, so access to a poison control center or other additional support will be provided. Your main job during a poisoning is to maintain airway, breathing, and circulation and to try to find out what substance the patient was exposed to, whether that be bottles on the ground or a syringe near the patient.

There are four main ways for a poison to enter the body, and those are inhalation, injection, ingestion, and absorption. Different poisons utilize different routes, and there will be different types of treatment for each route:

- *Inhalation* is when the patient breathes in the poisons. This is possible when the poison is gaseous, or suspended in air. Inhaled poisons can cause damage to the lung and respiratory system, as well as irritate exposed mucus membranes, such as the eyes and throat, and cause headache or dizziness. Depending on the poisons, patients may have seizures or an altered mental status. When treating a patient who has inhaled poison, they must be taken away from the source of the poison and may need to be given oxygen. With inhaled poisons, do not rely on pulse oximetry to indicate supplemental oxygen, as it is unreliable in this case. An important thing to note is that if a patient shows signs of poisoning through inhalation, that poison may still be in the air and the scene may not be safe. Call a specialty hazmat team, depending on local protocols.

- *Injection* is when a poison is deposited under the skin, most commonly by a needle or insect stinger. Symptoms of injected poison are altered mental status; weakness; chills; and, depending on the type and amount injected, unresponsiveness. The most important part of treating injected poisons is to rapidly transport and to bring any substances found on scene that could be the injected poison to the hospital.
- *Ingestion* is when a poison is consumed orally. Symptoms vary greatly, but oftentimes, there will be nausea and vomiting or some type of gastrointestinal discomfort. This is the most common route of poisoning and is particularly dangerous for infants and young children. With ingested poisons, age and weight greatly affect how potent the poison is to the patient, so you should take those values as a part of taking patient history. To treat a patient who has ingested a poison, make sure the airway remains clear if compromised by vomiting, and maintain breathing and circulation. Call poison control to understand how to better treat the patient. Some local protocols allow for the use of *activated charcoal*. Activated charcoal is an ingested medication which is meant to bind to the poison in the stomach before the poison is absorbed. However, it only works with a select few substances.
- *Absorption* is when a poison is absorbed transdermally or through contact with the skin. Symptoms of absorbed poisons are skin irritation or localized burns. To treat, you must first remove the source of the poison from the skin. If it is a dry poison or a powder, brush off the powder, and then, rinse the area of the skin with water for 15–20 minutes. If the poison is liquid, wash the skin with water for 15–20 minutes. If the affected area is the eyes, flush one eye with water or saline without contaminating the other. Make sure to decontaminate the patient and/or initially flush off the chemical prior to transport.

Each type of poison has different symptoms and characteristics, and you cannot know each and every one. Overall, a good general guideline when dealing with poisons is to remove patients from the poison, monitor and maintain ABC's, and call the poison control center if you do not know how to treat the patient.

Chapter Summary

Section "Endocrine Emergencies"
- The endocrine system regulates the production of hormones within the body.
- Glucose, or sugar, is essential for the body to function and, therefore, needs to be regulated carefully within the body.

Section "Environmental Emergencies"
- In order to survive and to work efficiently, the body has to maintain a state of homeostasis and has many different internal processes meant to maintain a stable internal environment.

Section "Abdominal Emergencies"
- The assessment of the abdomen involves palpation of all four quadrants and auscultating bowel sounds.
- Patients with acute abdominal pain always come with a potential for shock. Monitor your patient closely, and reassess vital signs regularly for hypotension or hypoxia.

Section "Poisons and Toxins"
- *Poisons* are any substances which chemically damage the body or body functions.
- Each type of poison has different symptoms and characteristics. Monitor and maintain ABCs, and call the poison control center if you do not know how to treat the patient.

Practice Questions
1. If a patient has been having a pain in their lower abdomen which has been slowly travelling toward their navel, what abdominal issue can be suspected?

   (a) Gallbladder infection
   (b) Appendicitis
   (c) Diverticulitis
   (d) Kidney stones

2. How are the amounts of insulin and glucose within the circulatory system related?

   (a) They are directly proportional.
   (b) They are inversely proportional.
   (c) They are unrelated.

3. You arrive on scene to a patient unconscious on the ground, as you assess them, you notice that their breath has a fruity scent. What emergency does this indicate?

   (a) Hypoglycemia
   (b) Appendicitis
   (c) Diabetic ketoacidosis

4. You arrive on scene to multiple people unresponsive and a carbon monoxide alarm going off. Through what route could you suspect these people were poisoned?

   (a) Injection
   (b) Absorption
   (c) Inhalation

Chapter 8
Trauma

Introduction

EMS calls that you will receive as a first responder will be organized into medical emergencies and trauma emergencies. The previous sections took you through the most common medical emergencies, and this section will cover traumatic injuries and related emergencies. Traumatic emergencies are very often the most shocking calls that you will be called on and are very diverse. They range from small broken fingers and sprained ankles to car crashes and far falls. However, despite the mechanism of injury, many of the same principles govern all traumatic injuries. Bleeding control, immobilization, and good airway management are the backbone of treating and assessing traumatic emergencies.

Kinematics of Trauma

Learning Objectives
Upon completing this section, you should be able to

- *understand the basic physics of trauma,*
- *identify laws of motion and energy transfer,*
- *infer the relationship of speed to injury,*
- *communicate principles of energy exchange.*

Kinematics of trauma is the study of how objects in motion are related to bodily injury. In this section, we will briefly discuss how physics plays a role in trauma before, during, and after an event. A basic understanding of kinematics is

C. Ventura et al., *The Emergency Medical Responder*, https://doi.org/10.1007/978-3-030-64396-6_8

prerequisite to thorough assessment and the assembly of a clinical suspicion index. With these kinematic tools, you'll be able to understand the importance of vehicle speed in a collision, the dangers of blunt force trauma, and how pedestrians respond to car strikes.

Isaac Newton's first law of motion tells us that an object in a resting state will remain at rest, unless acted upon by some external force. For example, an eight ball will likely remain in place until struck. The second law and the law of conservation of energy state that energy cannot be created nor destroyed, only changed and transformed, and that force can be described as mass multiplied by acceleration. Finally, the third law states that for every action that exists, there is an equal but opposite reaction. For example, if you lay this book on a table, there is a force pushing the book down onto the table (gravity) and a force up against the book so that the book does not fall through the table.

In all motor vehicle collisions, there is a minimum of three mini-collisions that occur rapidly:

1. Vehicle against another object that is still or in motion (i.e., car vs. tree)
2. Patient against the vehicle (i.e., the head vs. steering wheel)
3. Internal organs against cavity walls (i.e., the brain against the skull)

For a restrained patient wearing a seat belt, the patient comes to a stop when the vehicle stops. In the case of an unrestrained passenger, the patient will likely continue in motion at a continuous rate of speed until being halted by another object, such as the front windshield. In all types of collisions, there are the phases.

The *pre-event* phase encompasses all events and occurrences prior to the collision. This includes any preexisting medical illnesses that can affect a patient's prognosis, but not necessarily the kinematics of the event. The *event* phases include the three mini-collisions previously discussed. The *post-event* phase details all attempts of patient care and resuscitation.

It is important to understand that injury occurs due to an unideal transfer of kinetic energy.

We can express this mathematically as follows:

$$KE = 1/2 \; mv^2 \text{ or kinetic energy} = (0.5)(\text{mass})(\text{velocity})^2$$

To keep things simple, we'll use the terms *velocity* and *speed* and *mass* and *weight* interchangeably, although this is not technically true. If you look at the equation closely, you'll notice that one variable of the equation influences overall kinetic energy significantly, which is speed. This is because it's the value of speed squared. This means that the greatest indicator of injury is not necessarily the mass of the vehicle or the mass of the patient, but the speed at which the vehicle is going. Yes, this does mean that slowing down saves lives.

For adult patients, pedestrian vs. motor vehicle injuries occur in three phases:

1. Impact to the pelvis, hips, and lower extremities.
2. Torso rolling onto the hood of the vehicle (often combined with striking the windshield).

3. Patient falls to the ground, often head first.

For pediatric pedestrians striking motor vehicles, children often have a tendency to turn in toward the car. Three phases also occur here:

1. Impact to the upper body, sometimes the face.
2. Impact to the head as it strikes the top of the hood.
3. Patient falls to the ground, likely backward and head first.

Hemorrhaging

Learning Objectives
Upon completing this section, you should be able to

- *understand* the functions of different blood vessels within the circulatory system,
- *identify* the source of a hemorrhage by the pattern of bleeding,
- *infer* the type of treatment that may be used based on the severity of the hemorrhage,
- *communicate* to receiving medical personal as to whether the patient may have internal bleeding.

In EMS, seeing and treating different types of hemorrhages, or bleeding, are a common occurrence and will be a part of many trauma calls. Two overarching categories of hemorrhages are important to recognize and watch out for when responding to emergencies, internal and external bleeding.

External bleeding is when the hemorrhage directs blood outside of the body. This is the easiest category of hemorrhage to treat because the type and source of the bleeding are visible and readily accessible to the provider. It can be caused by any traumatic incident which causes a break in the skin, whether that be a piercing wound, an abrasion, or even a blunt force which splits the skin. Within this category, the type of hemorrhage can be classified by the source of the bleeding.

Arterial bleeding is when the hemorrhage occurs from one of the arteries in the body. The arteries are the blood vessels which carry oxygenated blood from the heart to the rest of the body and the heart muscle. Externally, arterial bleeding is indicated by spurting, bright red blood. Many times, the blood flow will pulse in time with the patient's heartbeat. Arterial bleeding is considered to be the most dangerous type of hemorrhage, because the patient is likely to bleed out very quickly.

Venous bleeding is when the hemorrhage occurs from one of the veins in the body. The veins carry deoxygenated blood back to the heart. Externally, venous bleeding is indicated by a steady flow of dark red blood. While this type of bleeding is still deadly if left untreated, it is slower than arterial bleeding.

Capillary bleeding is mostly superficial, with the hemorrhage stemming from capillaries. Capillaries are small vessels through which oxygen is diffused into surrounding tissue. This type of bleeding is not usually life-threatening and much easier to manage than the other two types of hemorrhages. It is indicated by a slow, oozing bleed.

Critical Skill: *Hemorrhage Control*
1. Apply appropriate PPE precautions, gloves and goggles at the minimum.
2. Apply direct pressure with a towel or gauze to the site of the bleeding.
3. If the bleeding does not stop, pack additional dressing. Never remove the first dressing, as this is critical for the clotting process.
4. If you suspect the bleeding is arterial and it is not easily resolved with direct pressure, apply a tourniquet.
5. Once the bleeding is controlled, raise the extremity if possible, administer high-flow oxygen, and observe closely for signs of shock.

Internal bleeding is when the hemorrhage occurs within the patient's body. Many times, this entails a compromised vessel bleeding into a bodily cavity, not visible to you as a responder. Even if it is not visible, internal bleeding is just as, if not more, dangerous than external bleeding, and there is no way to stop it in the field. Internal bleeding can be caused by blunt force trauma or even fractures internally nicking a vessel. For example, a broken femur can nick the femoral artery and can make a patient bleed out in minutes. It can be recognized sometimes by large areas of bruising around the affected area and by recognizing shock symptoms, which will be explained in the next chapter. Internal bleeding should be assumed when arriving on scene to a traumatic emergency, and you should always test for shock in your initial assessment.

Hypoperfusion (Shock)

Learning Objectives
Upon completing this section, you should be able to

- *understand* how hypoperfusion harms the body,
- *identify* different causes of hypoperfusion,
- *infer* how to treat different types of hypoperfusion based on their causes,
- *communicate* how to recognize hypoperfusion in a patient.

Hypoperfusion, commonly known as shock, occurs when there is an insufficient circulation of oxygenated blood. This means that oxygen is not being delivered to tissue essential for life and, left untreated, will lead to death. There are many different types of shock, each with unique causes, such as the following:

Anaphylactic shock is caused by the overdilation of blood vessels in reaction to an allergen, which means that there is not enough internal pressure to circulate blood.

Septic shock is a result of sepsis, a type of blood infection that affects the blood's ability to carry oxygen.

Cardiogenic shock occurs when there is a heart problem which prevents it from properly pumping blood.

There are more types of shock, but the one that you will be dealing with the most in a trauma setting is *hypovolemic* shock. Hypovolemic shock occurs when there is not enough fluid in the body for blood to properly circulate. This rarely occurs in a medical emergency when a patient has been gradually releasing fluids, for example, through vomiting and diarrhea, faster than they can replenish their fluid supply. This most commonly occurs in children and elderly. In terms of a trauma emergency, hypovolemic shock occurs acutely due to blood loss. For example, if there is a patient with arterial bleeding, whether external or internal, they no longer have enough blood to properly circulate oxygen throughout their body.

Recognizing shock as early as possible is important in giving effective treatment. One of the most easily recognizable signs is that the patient's skin will be cold and clammy and may appear pale. A certain combination of vital signs is also indicative of shock. That combination is low blood pressure, tachycardia, and tachypnea.

Managing shock in-field consists of three main steps. The patient should be given high-flow oxygen, be kept warm utilizing a blanket, and be rapidly transported. If possible, the cause of the shock should be managed. For example, if it is hypovolemic shock, treating the patient would include hemorrhage control.

Soft Tissue Injuries

Learning Objectives
Upon completing this section, you should be able to

- *understand* the function of the skin and how it is structured,
- *identify* different types of soft tissue injuries,
- *infer* whether or not an injury is life-threatening,
- *communicate* the severity of a burn on a patient.

Soft tissue injuries include injuries to the skin and mucous membranes on the body. This includes both injuries that lie on the surface of the skin and those that lie directly beneath, and they can be categorized accordingly.

To understand soft tissue injuries, it is important to understand the skin itself. The skin consists of three layers. The epidermis is the topmost layer of the skin. Its main job is to protect the body from the elements. The dermis is the second layer of the skin which contains hair follicles and sweat glands. The subcutaneous tissue is the bottommost layer, containing fat and blood vessels.

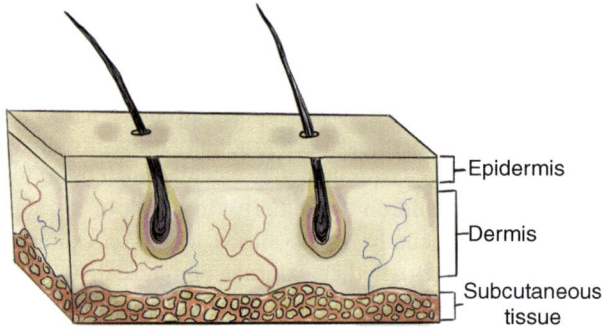

Open injuries are injuries that cause a break in the skin. There are four main types of injuries that fall in this category. The main aspects of these injuries to monitor in the field are hemorrhage control and preventing infection as much as the scene will allow.

A laceration is a cut which tears the skin. This injury is managed by hemorrhage control procedures, as previously described.

An abrasion is an injury which scraps only the top layers of the skin, like when a child scrapes his knee against concrete. As this injury is superficial and very rarely life-threatening, you will not have to treat it in the field and should not become distracted by the injury in the face of worse problems.

An avulsion occurs when two layers of the affected skin or membrane separate from each other. Never further separate the tissues. If the layers are still connected, the top layer will appear as a flap, which should be replaced on the patient before wrapping with gauze or performing any hemorrhage control procedures. Always bring completely avulsed pieces of skin, or tissue, to the hospital with the patient, wrapped with gauze. This is true with small pieces of skin as well as larger areas of tissue that may be amputated or removed from the body.

A penetrating wound is when the skin is pierced by a sharp object. Penetrating wounds tend to be deep and do a lot of internal damage. What you can do in that case is control external bleeding and transport. If whatever object that pierced the skin is still impaled within the body, never remove it, unless the placement of the object is preventing you from giving critical, lifesaving care, such as CPR. Leave the object in place, wrapping the site in gauze around the object to immobilize it so transport does not cause the object to do any more damage.

Closed injuries occur when the skin does not break, but there is still damage beneath the skin. There is not a way to treat these injuries in the field, but they should be monitored, and their possible effects, such as shock, should be treated. The main causes of closed injuries are blunt and crushing forces, with the greater the force, the worse the injuries. Contusions, or bruises, indicate bleeding under the skin and are a sign that there is internal damage to some degree. A hematoma is a large buildup of blood right under the skin, causing a large dark red area to form.

Crushing injuries require slightly different attention. If a body part is crushed by an object for a long time, over 4 hours, the patient could develop crush syndrome. This occurs when toxic waste from dying cells in the affected area builds up, so if the crushing force is released, that toxic waste would flood the body and be harmful, possibly even causing cardiac arrest. Crush syndrome has to be dealt with on an ALS level.

Burns are another type of soft tissue injury which are caused by the over-absorption of energy, whether that be thermal, electrical, or chemical energy. Burns can be classified by their source (thermal, electrical, or chemical) and depth.

First-degree burns only damage the epidermis. It is painful, but superficial and not immediately dangerous. The skin will be red and has no other physical differences. A light sunburn is an example of a first-degree burn.

Second-degree burns partially damage the dermis as well as the epidermis. Unlike with first-degree burns, the skin will start to blister and will be red or white. They will be even more painful than first-degree burns.

Third-degree burns are the most severe, penetrating through the entirety of the epidermis and dermis and sometimes damaging the subcutaneous tissue or underlying organs and tissue. The skin will not be red, but a white or charred brown. The site of the third degree burn may not be painful due to nerve damage, but severe burn will be surrounded with less severe burns, which will still cause the patient extreme pain.

When assessing the severity of burns and their dangers to the patient's life, it is important to be able to estimate how much of the body is burned. This is possible with two rules used to measure surface area. One rule, called the *rule of nines*, is that the palm of your hand is equal to one percent of the body's surface area and the rest of the body is split into multiples of 9% of the body's surface area.

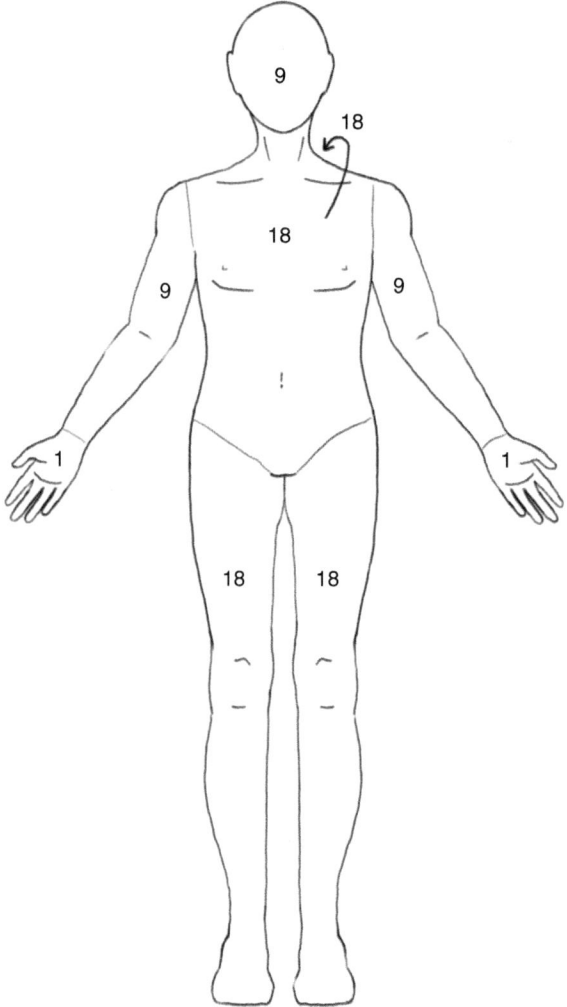

A patient with severe burns has burns covering 20 percent of their body or more, or any third-degree burn. These patients should be rapidly transported to specialized care. They should also be watched for shock, as burns lead to fluid loss, and hypothermia, as the temperature regulation role that the skin plays has been compromised. Moderate burns occur when 10–20 percent of the body is burned, and anything less is considered minor.

To treat burns, you must first remove the patient from the source of the burn. Then, start the patient on high-flow oxygen, and secure a dry, sterile dressing loosely over the burn site. Determine the severity of the burn and watch for shock and hypothermia.

Musculoskeletal Injuries

Learning Objectives
Upon completing this section, you should be able to,

- *understand* the causes of musculoskeletal injuries
- *identify* the different types of fractures,
- *infer* how to immobilize different types of injuries from a standardized procedure,
- *communicate* transportation decisions based on the patient's injuries.

Musculoskeletal injuries are a common emergency that you will respond to and can occur whenever excessive force is applied to the body. They can cause the patients a lot of pain and affect their mobility. This is why immobilization and transport have to be handled carefully in these cases and a good understanding of musculoskeletal injuries is vital.

Traumatic muscle injuries are common and not life-threatening to the patient. They are painful and can affect mobility, but further internal damage is not a risk, unlike with some skeletal injuries. There are two main types of muscle injuries that you will encounter as an EMT.

A *strain* is equivalent to a pulled muscle and occurs when a muscle or tendon is torn or overstretched. This causes bruising and swelling along the site of the injury as well as localized pain upon movement or palpation.

A *sprain* occurs when ligaments in a joint are torn due to overextension. There will be swelling, bruising, and pain at the affected joint. The patient will struggle using or putting pressure on the affected joint.

Common skeletal injuries are fractures, more commonly known as broken bones. There are many different types of fractures, each with a specific mechanism of injury attached.

First of all, the fracture can either be *open* (compound) or *closed* (simple). An open fracture is when a piece of bone breaks through the skin. A closed fracture occurs when the skin surrounding the injuries remains intact.

A *comminuted* fracture occurs when the bone is broken into multiple pieces, or fragments. This type of fracture is dangerous because those bone fragments can pierce and do damage to internal structures.

A *transverse* fracture occurs when a bone has a fracture running horizontally through it.

A *greenstick* fracture is a special case, as it most commonly occurs in children. As pediatric bones have more elasticity, sometimes, when excessive force is applied, they will bend and splinter instead of breaking clearly like the more brittle adult bones. This splintering fracture is a greenstick fracture.

Communicated   Transverse   Greenstick
Fracture   Fracture   Fracture

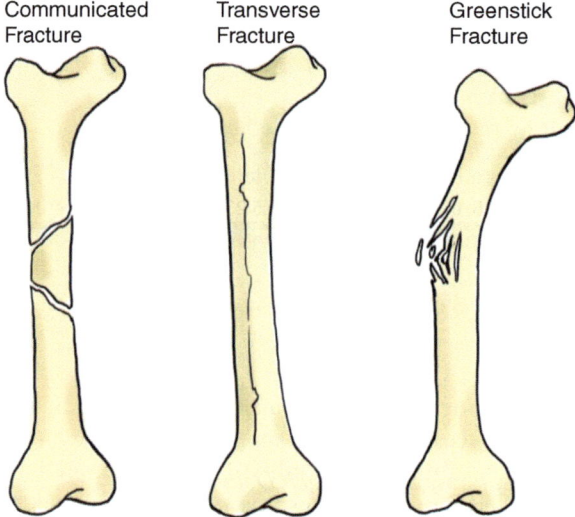

Another type of skeletal injury is a *dislocation*. This occurs when the ends of the bones involved in a joint break contact, for example, if the top of the humerous was popped out of the shoulder girdle. This injury is normally accompanied by torn ligaments in the joint and sometimes a fracture. Many times, dislocations may relocate back to its normal position in transport; however, the patient will still need medical attention due to associated injuries, like torn ligaments.

Treatment of musculoskeletal injuries in the field consists of immobilization in preparation for transport, as well as addressing any other symptoms the patient may have. For this, you will need to know how to use splints.

Critical Skill: *Long Bone Splinting*
- *Step 1:* Direct your partner to perform manual stabilization of the bone.
- *Step 2:* Assess circulatory, motor, and sensory function in the extremity.
- *Step 3:* Measure and place a splinting item such as a SAM splint or long wooden splint along the extremity such that it immobilizes the joint above and below the fractured bone.
- *Step 4:* Slide the securing devices such as triangular bandages under the extremity, and splint with minimal movement to the extremity.
- *Step 5:* Tightly tie or close the securing device to the extremity.
- *Step 6:* Reassess the circulatory, motor, and sensory function of the extremity, and if there is a negative chance in any of the areas, remove the splint and repeat the procedure.

Critical Skill: *Joint Splinting*
- *Step 1:* Direct your partner to perform manual stabilization of the bone.
- *Step 2:* Assess circulatory, motor, and sensory function in the extremity.
- *Step 3:* Measure and place a splinting item such as a SAM splint or long wooden splint along the extremity such that it immobilizes the bone above and below the fractured bone.
- *Step 4:* Slide the securing devices such as triangular bandages under the extremity, and splint with minimal movement to the extremity.
- *Step 5:* Tightly tie or close the securing device to the extremity.
- *Step 6:* Reassess the circulatory, motor, and sensory function of the extremity, and if there is a negative chance in any of the areas, remove the splint and repeat the procedure.

Critical Skill: *Triangular Bandage Application*
- *Step 1:* Have your partner or the patient stabilize the injured extremity.
- *Step 2:* Assess circulatory, motor, and sensory function in the extremity.
- *Step 3:* Tie a knot on the shortest corner of the triangular bandage, and place at the elbow of the injured extremity.
- *Step 4:* Place the end closest to the patient under the injured arm and on the shoulder of the injured extremity.
- *Step 5:* Place the remaining end over the injured arm and on the shoulder opposite to the injured extremity.
- *Step 6:* Secure the two ends together around the back of the neck with a safety pin or knot.
- *Step 7:* Apply a swath laterally around the patient and tie with a knot.
- *Step 8:* Reassess the circulatory, motor, and sensory function of the extremity, and if there is a negative chance in any of the areas, remove the sling and swath and repeat the procedure.

Critical Skill: *Application of a Traction Splint*
- *Step 1:* Assess circulatory, motor, and sensory function in the extremity.
- *Step 2:* Stabilize the extremity with one hand above and one below the area of the injury.
- *Step 3:* Direct your partner to apply the ankle hitch and take over manual inline traction of the extremity.
- *Step 4:* Place the splint under the legs and measure the traction splint to the appropriate length.

- *Step 5:* Apply the ischial strap to the patient on the upper thigh.
- *Step 6:* Attach the ankle hitch and pull mechanical traction till the patient reports pain relief. You partner can now release manual traction.
- *Step 7:* Secure the remaining support straps.
- *Step 8:* Reassess the circulatory, motor, and sensory function of the extremity, and if there is a negative chance in any of the areas, remove the sling and swath and repeat the procedure.
- *Step 9:* Secure the patient to a long backboard for transport.

Chapter Summary

Section "Kinematics of Trauma"
- The severity of trauma is dependent on the amount of force applied.
- For each vehicle collision, there are three mini-collisions, each with the potential to do harm to the body.

Section "Hemorrhaging"
- There are three main types of hemorrhaging, or bleeding. Arterial, venous, and capillary.
- Bleeding can happen either internally or external, and how you are able to control the bleeding is dependent on this and the hemorrhage type.

Section "Hypoperfusion (Shock)"
- Hypoperfusion, or shock, occurs when oxygenated blood is not adequately perfused within the body.
- There are many different kinds of shock, including anaphylactic, septic, and cardiogenic.

Section "Soft Tissue Injuries"
- The two categories of soft tissue injuries are open and closed. Open includes lacerations, avulsions, and abrasions. Closed includes bruises and crushing injuries.
- To assess a burn, you have to determine its severity, of which there are three levels, and how much of the body the burn covers, using the rule of nines.

Section "Musculoskeletal Injuries"
- Muscle injuries include strains and sprains.
- Skeletal injuries include many types of fractures, like transverse, comminuted, and greenstick, and dislocations.

Practice Questions

1. You arrive on scene to an adult patient who has spilled boiling water on themselves. Upon assessment, you note that the burn covers the entirety of the front of the patient's chest. What percent of the patient's body was burned?

   (a) 18%
   (b) 9%
   (c) 25%
   (d) 20%

2. While skydiving, a patient broke their tibia upon landing. Their tibia was broken into multiple pieces during the impact. What type of fracture do they have?

   (a) Transverse
   (b) Greenstick
   (c) Comminuted

3. A patient had a kitchen accident and has sustained a cut on their lower right forearm. The cut is oozing a dark red blood. What type of blood vessel did the patient cut?

   (a) Artery
   (b) Vein
   (c) Capillary

4. What type of shock occurs due to a loss of blood or fluid?

   (a) Cardiogenic shock
   (b) Septic shock
   (c) Anaphylactic shock
   (d) Hypovolemic shock

Chapter 9
The Trauma Assessment

Learning Objectives
This chapter will teach you how to thoroughly assess a traumatic patient using the guidelines established by the NREMT and will coach you in preparing for the psychomotor exam.

Part 1: Scene Size-Up

1. *Take proper PPE precautions.* Say: "BSI is my scene-safe?" Do: Don appropriate PPE, and wait for proctor response.
2. *Determine mechanism of injury and/or nature of illness.* Say: "It appears that the MOI/NOI is _____, is that correct?"
3. *Determine number of patients.* Say: "Is this my only patient?" or "Number of patients: _____."
4. *Request additional resources if necessary.* Say: "I will/will not request for additional resources at this time" Think: Are ABCs compromised in any way?
5. *Consider C-spine stabilization.* Say: "I will/will not have my partner take C-spine precautions." Think: Is a spinal injury likely? Did the patient fall from over three times their height? When in doubt: Apply a collar.

© The Author(s), under exclusive license to Springer Nature
Switzerland AG 2021
C. Ventura et al., *The Emergency Medical Responder*,
https://doi.org/10.1007/978-3-030-64396-6_9

Part 2: Primary Survey

6. *Verbalize general impression.*
7. *Determine level of responsiveness.* Think: What does this patient score on the AVPU scale?
8. *Determine immediate life threats/chief complaint.* Think: Is there major bleeding? A sucking chest wound? Do: Conduct a rapid blood sweep.
9. *Check airway.* Think: Is it patent? Do: Perform jaw thrust, insert oral adjunct, ventilate, and suction if appropriate.
10. *Check breathing.* Think: What is the rate, quality, and depth of breathing? Do: Oxygen therapy if indicated.
11. *Check circulation.* Think: Are pulses equal and regular? Fast or slow? What is the skin's color, temperature, and capillary refill status? Do: Treat any major bleeding, and treat for shock if indicated.
12. *Make a transport decision.* Think: Does the patient need to be transported immediately? To what type of facility?

Part 3: History Taking

13. *Obtain baseline vital signs.* Think: Does the patient's pulse rate, respiratory rate, blood pressure, or O2 saturation tell us anything?
14. *Obtain a sample history* Think: Is the patient able to tell us this information? How about a bystander? Sometimes, a history is unobtainable.

Part 4: Secondary Survey

15. *Assess the head.* Palpate frontal to occipital; is there any DCAP-BTLS? Are the pupils equal and reactive to light? Is there blood or CSF coming out of the ears, nose, or mouth? Is the airway still patent?
16. *Assess the neck.* Is the trachea midline or shifted? Is there any jugular venous distention? Is there any cervical tenderness or step-offs?
17. *Assess the chest.* Are the clavicles intact? Check the sternum in a chopping motion. Is there any paradoxical movement, chest flail segments, or crepitus? Is the xiphoid process present? How are the lung sounds?

18. *Assess the abdomen/pelvis.* Palpate all four quadrants. Do you notice any distention, guarding, rigidity, or grimace? Are bowel sounds normal? Is the pelvis stable? Is a priapism present?
19. *Assess lower extremities.* Is there any DCAP-BTLS? Is there normal circulatory, motor, sensory, and distal function in each leg?
20. *Assess upper extremities.* Is there any DCAP-BTLS? Is there normal circulatory, motor, sensory, and distal function in each arm?
21. *Assess posterior lumbar, thorax, and buttocks.*

Part 5: Reassessment
22. *Verbalize reassessment.* How and when will you reassess your patient?

Chapter 10
The Medical Assessment

Learning Objectives
This chapter will teach you how to thoroughly assess a medical patient using the guidelines established by the NREMT and will coach you in preparing for the psychomotor exam.

Part 1: Scene Size-Up
1. *Take proper PPE precautions*. Say: "BSI is my scene-safe?" Do: Don appropriate PPE, and wait for proctor response.
2. *Determine mechanism of injury and/or nature of illness*. Say: "It appears that the MOI/NOI is _____, is that correct?"
3. *Determine number of patients*. Say: "Is this my only patient?" or "Number of patients: _____."
4. *Request additional resources if necessary*. Say: "I will/will not request for additional resources at this time" Think: Are ABCs compromised in any way?
5. *Consider C-spine stabilization*. Say: "I will/will not have my partner take C-spine precautions." Think: Is a spinal injury likely? Did the patient fall from over three times their height? When in doubt: Apply a collar; however, most medical patients do **not** need one.

C. Ventura et al., *The Emergency Medical Responder*, https://doi.org/10.1007/978-3-030-64396-6_10

Part 2: Primary Survey

6. *Verbalize general impression.*
7. *Determine level of responsiveness.* Think: What does this patient score on the AVPU scale?
8. *Determine immediate life threats/chief complaint.*
9. *Check airway.* Think: Is it patent? If the patient is talking to you, it is!
10. *Check breathing.* Think: What is the rate, quality, and depth of breathing? Do: Oxygen therapy if indicated.
11. *Check circulation.* Think: Are pulses equal and regular? Fast or slow? What is the skin's color, temperature, and capillary refill status? Do: Treat any major bleeding, and treat for shock if indicated.
12. *Make a transport decision.* Think: Does the patient need to be transported immediately? To what type of facility?

Part 3: History Taking

13. *Obtain baseline vital signs.* Think: Does the patient's pulse rate, respiratory rate, blood pressure, or O2 saturation tell us anything?
14. *Obtain a sample history.* Think: Is the patient able to tell us this information? How about a bystander? Sometimes, a history is unobtainable.
15. *Obtain an OPQRST.* Think: What are our clinical suspicions?

Part 4: Secondary Survey

16. Assess affected organ system/region.

Part 5: Reassessment

17. *Verbalize reassessment.* How and when will you reassess your patient?
18. *Provide accurate report.* Summarize all findings and interventions.

Chapter 11
Special Considerations

Introduction

Throughout the book and throughout most of EMS training, you are taught how to treat illness in the context of a healthy, adult individual. However, this is not always, in fact is rarely ever, the case. There are many different types of ways that patients can deviate from the training standard, and how to cater your method of treatment toward each of these ways will be covered in this chapter. Of course, you cannot know and cater toward every single population, but this chapter will give you a general overview of how treatment differs for geriatric patients, pediatric patients, and patients with impairments.

Patients with Impairments

Learning Objectives
Upon completing this section, you should be able to

- *understand* how to transport patients with mobility impairment,
- *identify* possible risks a patient may have due to their specific condition,
- *infer* how to cater treatment to each patient,
- *communicate* with each patient respectfully and appropriately.

Patients with physical impairments can range from those with sensory issues to those with mobility issues or chronic conditions.

Sensory impairment refers to patients who have problems with their hearing and/ or sight. When treating these patients, it is really important that communication is

C. Ventura et al., *The Emergency Medical Responder*,
https://doi.org/10.1007/978-3-030-64396-6_11

maintained. For those that are vision impaired, make sure that you let the patient know who you are, where you are, and what you are doing throughout the call. When walking with the patient, make them aware of any obstacles in their path. For those that are hearing impaired, always stay in their eyeline, and when speaking, face the patient, speaking slowly but without any exaggeration. If they are able to read lips, this will be helpful; however, only a small population can fully read lips. If they use sign language and have a friend or family member who can interpret, bring them in the ambulance, or request a translator for when you arrive at the receiving facility. For both types of impairments, bring any assisting equipment, such as glasses, hearing aids, or canes, with you to the hospital. Always alert the receiving facility if and when a translator may be needed.

If a patient has a condition that impairs mobility, assist in transportation, and bring any equipment, such as wheelchairs or walkers, with you to the hospital. More serious conditions that require equipment attached to the body to be maintained, such as feeding tubes or catheters, vary greatly. In these instances, transport cautiously, and if available, allow a caretaker to assist you.

Bariatric patients are patients who suffer from *obesity*, or an excess of body fat. From a transport perspective, some counties have special bariatric ambulances or equipment while others do not. One of the most important parts about transporting bariatric patients is to coordinate all lifts and moves with the other providers and ask for the opinion of the patient. This will prevent the patient becoming injured, as too much strain on the joints of a bariatric patient from transporting could do the patient serious injury. When communicating with the patient, be respectful at all times, and treat the patient with dignity.

Different medical assistance devices require different maintenance. If you have a patient with medical technology assistance, don't touch it unless necessary, and if you need to handle it, ask a caregiver, the patient, or medical direction for help. There are many types of devices that lie beneath the skin that you will not have to manage directly; however, some are a little more complicated:

- *Tracheostomy tube* is a tube that is placed in the patient's throat to help them breath. This tube can get clogged, obstructing the patient's airway. If this happens, you can suction it using either the patient's own suction device or placing the suction in the tube, no more than 2 inches, and suctioning for no more than 10 seconds.
- *External defibrillator vests*, which monitor the patient's heart, delivering a shock if necessary, should be kept on at all times, unless they are actively interfering with a lifesaving procedure.

Aneurotypical Impairments

Autism spectrum disorder (*ASD*) is a widely varied developmental disorder which can affect the patient's social interaction and, therefore, how you communicate with the patient. Treat this patient as you would any other, except watch their body language as you approach and interact. Try not to overwhelm them by only having one provider approach them at a time while maintaining a calm, eye-level stance.

Down syndrome is a genetic disorder which affects mental development and the patient's physiology. Approach this patient just as we discussed previously with autistic patients, and remember to treat this patient overall as you would any other. The physiological changes may change the way you treat the patient. For example, patients with Down syndrome have different upper respiratory passageways, meaning that adjuncts will be difficult to place and may not be an option depending on the patient. Patients with Down syndrome are at risk for many health issues, specifically heart problems and epilepsy, which are important to keep in mind during your assessment.

Understand that adult patients who are aneurotypical are capable and competent adults and in most cases are independent. Avoiding patronizing language is conducive to high-quality care. Always ask before rendering assistance, and respect their decisions, always.

Geriatric Considerations

Learning Objectives
Upon completing this section, you should be able to

- *understand* the physiological state of the geriatric population,
- *identify* possible elder abuse from physical signs,
- *infer* how to comfortable transport elderly patients,
- *communicate* with the patient appropriately.

We have already discussed many of the physiological changes that occur once a person reaches the older adult stage of life (greater than 65 years of age) in the human development chapter. In older adulthood, the body, including every organ system, becomes more at risk for chronic diseases. This is the stage of life where cardiac conditions such as congestive heart failure and myocardial infarctions become more common. The respiratory system weakens, and the endocrine system becomes more at risk for diabetes. The skin becomes more delicate and breaks more easily.

The skeletal system also goes through massive changes. As a person reaches the last stage of life, the bones become more brittle and are easier to break. That is why a broken pelvis, while being very rare among younger populations, is common among the geriatric population and should be carefully checked for during the patient assessment. A simple slip in the shower or fall down the stairs, while resulting in a minor bruise or contusion for younger patients, can result in serious skeletal injuries in older adults. Not only do these injuries happen more often, but also they take longer to heal, making the patient at risk for further complications. Another common change in the skeletal system is spinal curvature. This needs to be taken into consideration when transporting and backboarding a patient. Additional padding should be used for these patients.

Spinal curvature is not the only condition that can affect the transportation of geriatric patients. Changes in the musculoskeletal system can affect the patient's mobility, and many of the geriatric patients you treat may use a walking aid or wheelchair. You may need to assist the patient in moving to or from the ambulance.

Another consideration that you will need to consider when caring for geriatric patients has to do with the compromised nervous system that some geriatric patients possess. As with the rest of the body, the nervous system also weakens in older patients, causing geriatric patients to have slower reflexes, confusion, and other presenting conditions such as dementia. While the patient may have a compromised mental state, it is important to not treat the patient like a child or assume that they have a compromised mental state. If they have a caregiver, communicate with them, and allow them to help, as they best understand the patient, but communicate with the patient as well throughout the call.

Many elderly patients will have a caregiver or live primarily in a nursing home because of the previously discussed physiological and mental changes occurring. This reliance on others puts the patients in a vulnerable position, opening up the possibility of *elder abuse*, defined as physical, psychological, or financial abuse by a caregiver or family member. Look for unusual bruising on the patient, such as bruises in multiple stages of healing or in uncommonly injured places. Also, look for signs of neglect, such as malnourishment or a lack of hygiene. These signs can help you identify elder abuse, and you should follow local protocols in reporting the incident.

Pediatric Considerations

Learning Objectives
Upon completing this section, you should be able to

- *understand* how to properly assess a pediatric patient,
- *identify* when a child is going into shock,
- *infer* how to adapt transportation to support the child's airway,
- *communicate* with the child and caregiver equally.

The different stages of pediatric development and their attached physiological and psychological changes were outlined in the human development chapter. This section will speak about specific considerations you need to take when treating and communicating within a pediatric emergency.

For example, there are certain illnesses that manifest specifically in children or differently in children. An important one is hypoperfusion (shock). In pediatric emergencies, blood pressure is not as good of an indicator as to whether the child is in shock or not. In adults, shock progresses gradually, and signs such as blood pressure parallel that progression. However, in children, their blood pressure will plateau and then suddenly drop, seeming stable but then progressing rapidly into severe hypoperfusion. This is why it is very important to continuously monitor children involved in traumatic emergencies. Also, children can progress into shock from certain illnesses that make them vomit excessively. If they are excreting more fluid than they are taking in, the pediatric anatomy does not have enough reserves to compensate.

Pediatric average heart rates and blood pressures differ, and those rates can be found in the human development section.

Another illness that can be found primarily in pediatric cases is a *febrile seizure*. This is a seizure normally occurring in infants that is caused by a high fever due to illness or infection.

Pediatric patients are susceptible to respiratory compromise, due to illness and the shape of their airway due to the size of their heads in proportion to the rest of their bodies. This is important to understand when transporting a pediatric patient and positioning their airway. Raise the child's shoulders about an inch off the ground when they are lying on a flat surface using a towel or pillow.

Airway obstructions are common in pediatric patients due to infection, such as croup and epiglottitis, and due to children placing small objects in their mouths. They are also common due to asthma, as discussed in the respiratory chapter.

In general, you must use the *Pediatric Assessment Triangle* to assess pediatric patients.

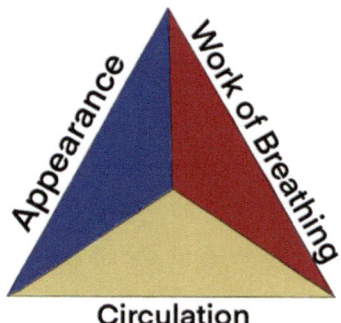

Circulation

When assessing appearance, you are looking at the child's activity levels and if they have good muscle tone. You will also assess if they can adequately interact with you by seeing if they have an abnormal gaze or speech pattern.

When assessing work of breathing, you will see if their respiration is irregular, if they show accessory muscle use, or if they have abnormal lungs.

With circulation, you will assess their pulse and whether their skin is mottled or cyanotic.

One of the most important parts of managing a pediatric emergency is communication. Do not lie to the child; try to gain their trust. It is important to communicate what is going on to both the child and the family, who may also need your support, and to not leave either out. If a caregiver is calm, they may be able to help you calm and gain the trust of the child.

Chapter Summary

Section "Patients with Impairments"
- Patients with physical impairments can range from those with sensory issues to those with mobility issues or chronic conditions.

Section "Geriatric Considerations"
- In older adulthood, the body, including every organ system, becomes more at risk for chronic diseases.
- As a person reaches the last stage of life, the bones become more brittle and are easier to break.

Section "Pediatric Considerations"
- There are certain illnesses that manifest specifically in children or differently in children.
- One of the most important parts of managing a pediatric emergency is communication.

Practice Questions

1. What type of seizure is most common in infants?

   (a) Complex partial seizure.
   (b) Febrile seizure.
   (c) Generalized tonic-clonic seizure.
   (d) There is no seizure specific to infants.

2. Why is backboarding more difficult for geriatric patients?

   (a) Increased discomfort
   (b) A decreased range of motion
   (c) Visual and auditory issues
   (d) Spinal curvature

3. Utilizing the Pediatric Assessment Triangle, what are you checking for while assessing appearance?

   (a) The child's skin tone
   (b) The child's work of breathing
   (c) The child's emotional stability
   (d) The child's activity level and muscle tone

Chapter 12
Principles of Death and Dying

Introduction

Many people join EMS with the goal of helping people and saving lives. EMS professionals save many thousands of lives per year, but it is important to know in advance that not all of your patients will survive. This is inevitable, and you should not see it as a negative reflection on yourself or your skills. Rather, you must learn to accept this fact and keep in mind not only those few patients you lose but also the many whose lives you have saved. Death is a concept that we often struggle with and often distance ourselves from. However, you will unfortunately face death at some point in either your personal or professional life. The emotions that come with experiencing death up close can be monumental. As a first responder, it is important that you understand how death affects not only you as a provider but also a patient's family and friends. In this chapter, you will learn about the psychological effects of a patient's death and how to deal with them, as well as how to console and interact with a patient's family and friends.

> **Learning Objectives**
> Upon completing this section, you should be able to
>
> - *understand* the emotional effects of death on the first responder,
> - *identify* the four stages of the grieving process,
> - *infer* what someone may be feeling after the death of a loved one,
> - *communicate* that a patient has died to their loved ones.

One of the most common feelings associated with death is grief. Everyone experiences grief at some point in their lives, and as such, it is important that we explain

C. Ventura et al., *The Emergency Medical Responder*, https://doi.org/10.1007/978-3-030-64396-6_12

and understand grief through a psychological lens. You have probably heard of the theory of the five stages of grief, originally proposed by Dr. Elizabeth Kübler-Ross in her book *On Death and Dying*. Here, they are in detail:

The Grieving Process
- Denial: In this stage, grievers may reject the events which are causing them to grieve, even substituting false realities.
- Anger: Grievers may lash out at those around them, including healthcare providers, and will seek to lay blame for the tragedy on some person or event.
- Bargaining: Grievers may try to negotiate or "trade" for the life of their loved one or even simply for more time with them.
- Depression: This stage is characterized by lack of interest and reduced socialization. The griever may question the purpose of life or ask what the point of life is if death is inevitable.
- Acceptance: This is the final stage of the grieving process and is characterized by the stabilization of a griever's emotional state. Eventually, they should be able to come to terms with their loved one's death and continue to live a normal life.

These five stages are by no means universal. Everyone experiences grief in different ways, and grievers may skip stages or spend most of their time in a single stage. In addition, the stages can be experienced in any order, and it is possible to repeat stages. Confront each situation as it comes, and do your best to be gentle and comforting.

Eventually, the time will come when you, in your capacity as a healthcare provider, must inform a loved one of a patient's death. This is a difficult process for both you and the loved one and should be approached with care. When delivering the news to a loved one, it is always preferable to speak to them in person, unless distance or some other factor makes this impossible. Additionally, try to speak to only a single person, allowing them to tell the rest of their friends and family about their loved one's death. Use plain language, and say unequivocally that the patient is dead. Avoid terms like "passed away" or "no longer with us," as these phrases can be confusing and unclear to people who are experiencing a catastrophic loss. Make it clear that everything possible was done to help save the patient. If the loved ones would like to see the patient, you should remove life support devices, clean the patient, and cover them with a sheet.

The recommendations above are by no means a set-in-stone protocol. No one is better equipped to deal with a situation than the first responder in that situation, and thus, you should use your best judgment and approach the task with care and empathy. No matter what, be supportive, and attempt to sympathize with friends and family while keeping cultural differences in mind.

Chapter 13
Psychiatric Emergencies

Introduction

In EMS, we often focus on the physical body of a patient and oftentimes overlook the mind of the patient. Many people may think that it's not that important, but a psychiatric condition can be just as dangerous as an abdominal laceration or traumatic brain injury. You will learn why this is the case in this chapter. We will also discuss how to assess and properly treat a patient with a psychiatric condition or illness.

Learning Objectives
Upon completing this section, you should be able to

- *understand* the importance of acknowledging a psychiatric condition,
- *identify* the signs and symptoms of a psychiatric emergency,
- *infer* what a psychiatric patient's point of view may be,
- *communicate* with a psychiatric patient in an understanding manner.

Behavioral or psychiatric emergencies can vary greatly in severity from abnormal behavior to suicidal ideation and attempts. Some of the other common psychiatric emergencies include depression and panic attacks. Just like any other condition, we must perform an assessment and uncover it by looking at the patient's signs and symptoms. Psychiatric emergencies are a bit different from cardiovascular or respiratory emergencies in that we primarily perform our assessment via asking the patient or the patient's family and friends questions. You may want to ask questions as to how the patient is feeling or ask a family member about their normal behavior to establish a baseline. One should also take into consideration anything that may increase the likelihood that there may be a psychiatric condition such as the death of

© The Author(s), under exclusive license to Springer Nature
Switzerland AG 2021
C. Ventura et al., *The Emergency Medical Responder*,
https://doi.org/10.1007/978-3-030-64396-6_13

a loved one, loss of a job, or recent diagnosis or a major illness. Take notes throughout the entire call on the patient's mood and activity levels and whether their thoughts are coherent or unorganized.

Psychiatric disorders are classified into two categories. *Organic* disorders are caused by a physiological malfunction of the nervous system. Many of the illnesses causing an altered mental status that we have previously discussed fall into this category, like hypoglycemia or strokes. Another example of this type of disorder is Alzheimer's disease, which you may see in a patient history.

The other type of psychiatric disorder is a *functional* disorder, where the physiological root of the disorder cannot be found. Most anxiety disorders fall into this category. This includes disorders like PTSD and social anxiety. Other disorders, such as schizophrenia, also are included in this category.

When treating and caring for a psychiatric patient, you should also keep in mind your safety and the safety of others. Always remember that scene safety is of utmost importance, and if the scene is not safe, do not enter. It is important to keep in mind your positioning in the room or building. You want to ensure that you have a clear path to the exit. Restraints typically are a last resort but can be used if the patient is a possible threat to you, others, or themselves upon approval by medical direction.

An emergency where one may need to consider using restraints is when the patient is in a state of excited delirium. This is categorized by irrational and agitated behavior. This does not explicitly mean that the patient is dangerous or requires restraint, but is something to look out for when taking a psychiatric call.

Critical Skill: *Application of Patient Restraints*
- *Step 1*: Have one partner maintain communication with the patient.
- *Step 2*: Have four people approach the patient each on a different side, and each person will be assigned one limb.
- *Step 3*: Move in quickly, and have each person restrain their assigned limb as directed by medical control.
- *Step 4*: Secure the restraints used on the patient to the stretcher.

When treating a psychiatric emergency, there are various legal and ethical considerations to consider. Just because a patient has a psychiatric condition or illness doesn't mean you no longer need to obtain consent. In order to treat a patient without given consent, you must determine that they are incapable of making decisions such as in the case of an altered mental status or that they are a threat to themselves or others. In this case, most protocols require that you request law enforcement and call for approval from medical direction.

Considerations for Radio Communications
- Be honest and truthful when talking with the patients.
- Maintain a reasonable distance, and avoid unnecessary physical contact with the patient.
- Make use of friends and family not only for getting information but also for the comfort of the patient.
- Remain calm even if the patient is aggravated or arguing with you.
- Establish a line of trust, and encourage the patient to open up about his or her feelings and emotions.

Chapter Summary

- Psychiatric conditions can be very dangerous and should be treated as such while making appropriate changes in your assessment to be more focused on the patient's mind via conversation with not only the patient but also their friends and family.

Practice Questions
1. What category of psychiatric emergency does an altered mental status secondary to hypoglycemia fall into?

   (a) Functional
   (b) Organic
   (c) Neither

2. When is the only time that physical restraints are even considered?

   (a) When the patient is agitated
   (b) When a patient is being verbally abusive
   (c) When a patient is a threat to themselves or others
   (d) Whenever a patient enters the ambulance

3. What is a consideration you should **not** make while a patient is having a psychiatric emergency?

   (a) Avoid unnecessary physical contact.
   (b) Speak loudly and close to the patient.
   (c) Speak quietly and calmly.
   (d) Be honest with the patient.

Chapter 14
Obstetrics and Gynecology

Introduction

This chapter will teach you how to deliver a baby and the different considerations that you will need to take in regard to both the delivering patient and the neonate. You will be a part of one of the most important moments in your patient's life, and you need to know how to treat the situation seriously and with care. This chapter will also touch on other gynecological emergencies and how they should be treated as well.

> **Learning Objectives**
> Upon completing this section, you should be able to
>
> - *understand* the principles of labor and delivery,
> - *identify* different complications during delivery,
> - *infer* the importance of emotional support for the patient during the described processes,
> - *communicate* with the patient respectfully throughout gynecological emergencies.

Pregnancy is the period of time where a *fetus*, an unborn child, develops and both the parent and the fetus go through immense physiological changes. A complete pregnancy, also known as complete gestation, is supposed to be 38 to 40 weeks long. This time period is split into three trimesters, each being about 3 months long. When dealing with a pregnant patient, the trimester or the length of pregnancy is a question that should be asked and documented. To understand those changes, one first needs to know a few terms and body structures. First of all, an unfertilized egg,

C. Ventura et al., *The Emergency Medical Responder*,
https://doi.org/10.1007/978-3-030-64396-6_14

before the egg becomes a fetus, is called an *ovum*. The fetus is held in the *uterus* for the duration of the pregnancy surrounded by a cushioning fluid called *amniotic fluid*, held in the amniotic sac. The fetus is attached to the mother through the placenta and the umbilical cord. The *placenta* is attached to the top of the uterine wall, and it transfers nutrients from the parent to the fetus and filters out waste. The *umbilical cord* attaches the fetus to the placenta. The opening of the uterus is the *cervix*, and that connects the uterus to the birth canal, which is called the *vagina*. These structures all play a part in pregnancy, labor, and delivery.

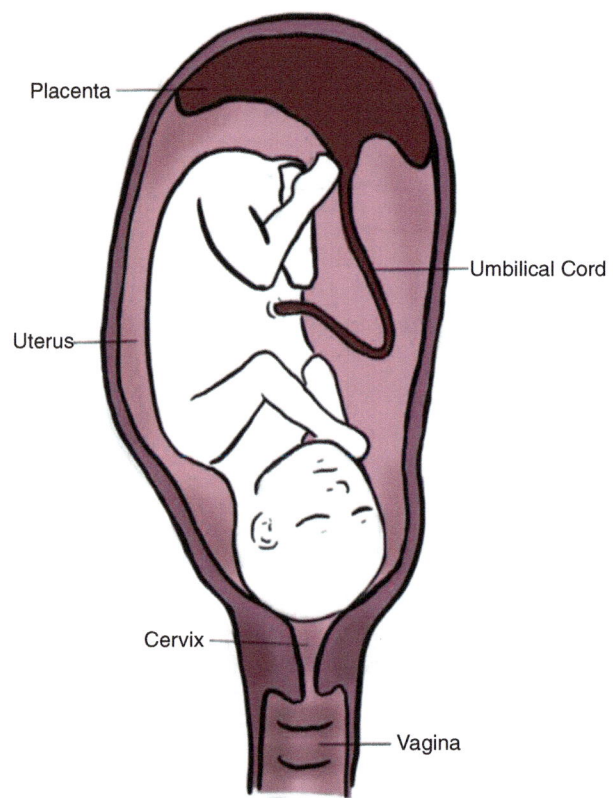

Labor

The process of labor is when the pregnancy ends and the body prepares to deliver the child. It starts with the dilation of the cervix and ends with a completed delivery. There are three main stages of labor, each representing a different step in the delivery of a child, and each EMS provider should be able to recognize them.

Stage 1 begins when the cervix starts to dilate. This will be evident because the mother will start having *contractions*. Either the mother will let you know that they are occurring (because I guarantee she will be acutely aware of the fact) or you can feel the tension of the muscles by placing your hand on the mother's abdomen. These contractions will initially be far apart, but the time between contractions, or the *interval time*, will steadily decrease throughout this stage. It is important to time the contractions from the beginning of one to the beginning of the next. Delivery is imminent once the interval time is 2 minutes or less. This stage ends once the cervix is fully dilated.

Stage 2 begins once the baby enters the birth canal and ends once the baby has been delivered. This process is the one an EMS provider will be involved in, and the steps on how to deliver the baby will be discussed later.

Stage 3 begins once the baby has been born and ends with the delivery of the placenta. This process is also called afterbirth.

Delivery

The first part of delivering a child is to determine whether or not delivery is imminent. Throughout your encounter with the patient, you should be timing their contractions. As mentioned earlier, if the contraction interval is less than 2 minutes, you should begin to prepare to deliver the baby in the field, barring any complications. Other signs that delivery is imminent are if there is blood show (blood-streaked mucus from the vagina); the amniotic sac has ruptured; or, for active delivery, there is crowning. *Crowning* is when the top of the baby's head is visible at the entrance to the vagina. To assess the presence of these signs, you need to visually, not physically, inspect the vagina. Do not touch the genital area except during delivery.

If you have determined that the delivery is imminent and there are no complications, you will have to deliver in the field. At this point, do not let the mother leave or go to the restroom. Each ambulance or station should be equipped with an OB kit containing all of the equipment that you will need for delivery in the field. This should include PPE such as goggles, gloves, and maybe a gown. It will also include materials such as towels or sheets to place under the patient during delivery. To aid the delivery, it will include a scalpel or scissors, gauze, and umbilical cord clamps. Finally, there will be the equipment needed to care for the baby immediately after the birth.

Place a sheet or towel under the patient, and use pillows under the patient's hips to elevate them about 2 inches, and ask the patient to spread their legs. Once you see crowning, delivery has begun. Support the head as it is delivered, and allow it to rotate sideways naturally, as this will allow the first shoulder to be delivered. As the head delivers, feel around the neck to check and see if the umbilical cord has wrapped around the baby's neck. If this occurs, use two fingers placed under the cord at the base of the baby's neck, and gently slip the cord over the baby's head. If the cord is too tight to slip over the head, use two clamps on the cord 2 inches apart, and cut the cord between them. Once this is clear, guide the baby's head downward to deliver the upper shoulder, and you may need to lightly guide the head up to deliver the lower shoulder. The rest of the body should deliver smoothly after the shoulders are delivered.

After the baby is delivered, make sure to clear the baby's airways, suctioning with a bulb syringe that can be found in the OB kit. You may need to tap the bottom of the baby's foot to facilitate breathing. If breathing does not start after 15 seconds of stimulation, start to resuscitate the newborn. Then, if you haven't already done so, clap the umbilical cord about 6 inches away from the patient, placing two clamps 2–4 inches apart and cutting between the clamps. Obtain an Apgar score, a system used to assess neonates after birth.

	0 Points	1 Point	2 Points
Appearance	Blue/pale	Blue extremities, pink core	Pink
Pulse	Absent	<100bpm	>100bpm
Grimace	Limp	Some flexion of arms and legs	Pulls away
Activity	Absent	Flexed arms and legs	Active movement
Respirations	Absent	Slow and irregular	Strong crying

If no emergency procedures, like airway management, need to be performed on the newborn, wrap them in a blanket and place the baby with the patient. By this time, you may resume transport while delivering the placenta, which you should bring to the hospital along with the umbilical cord. Once the placenta is delivered, which should not take more than 30 minutes, place a gauze pad over the vagina and massage the patient's abdomen to help slow bleeding. Monitor and manage both the patient's and the newborn's vitals and ABCs.

Complications in Labor and Delivery
As a general rule, if a delivery does not appear to be normal, which we will discuss further later, do not deliver, and transport immediately. If the delivery is already in progress, place the patient on all fours to help delay the birth. If a pregnant patient shows other issues, such as hypertension or excessive bleeding, place the patient in a recovery position on their left side and transport. However, now, we will cover some specific complications that can occur.

Premature delivery is when delivery begins before 36 weeks of gestation. Ask the patient when they are due during the initial assessment, and if they are a confirmed premature delivery, be prepared for the baby to require intensive care and resuscitation upon delivery.

Postterm delivery is when delivery begins after 42 weeks of gestation. This puts the mother and the neonate at risk and increases the patient's chances of needing a C-section. Ask the patient when they are due and if their doctor has identified any problems with the neonate.

Spina bifida occurs when a portion of the spinal cord is not contained within the vertebrae making up the spine of the neonate. This should have been identified prior to delivery by the patient's doctor. Once delivered, cover the protrusion with agonist dressing under an occlusive dressing, and keep the baby warm, by either blankets or being held. Transport with caution.

Miscarriage occurs when the neonate has died prior to delivery. This can be recognized by a green or brown, foul-smelling fluid being excreted by the vagina. If delivery occurs and the baby shows signs of decay, do not resuscitate and focus on comforting the patient.

Prolapsed cord is when, instead of crowning, the first thing to present in the vagina is the umbilical cord. Do not deliver or cut the cord. Cover the cord with a moist dressing, and transport on all fours, as mentioned previously. Insert your fingers under the cord to gently push the baby's head away from the cord, so their blood supply is not cut prematurely.

Limb presenting occurs when, instead of crowning, the first thing to present in the vagina is one of the neonate's limbs. Do not deliver, but transport the patient on all fours.

Breech delivery occurs when the fetus is backward in the uterus, meaning the first thing to present is the baby's buttocks. Deliver as you would normally, but call for ALS support. The delivery should progress smoothly until reaching the head, which will normally deliver facedown. As the head delivers, place your fingers into the vagina against the baby's face in a v shape around the airway to protect the airway during delivery.

Placenta previa occurs when the placenta forms over the cervical opening. This means that the baby cannot be delivered, as the placenta is blocking the opening of the birth canal. This condition should be identified early on in the pregnancy and requires rapid transport.

Placental abruption occurs when the placenta tears prematurely from the uterine wall. This will result in excessive bleeding from the vagina and could be potentially lethal for both the fetus and the patient. If you notice excessive vaginal bleeding from a pregnant patient, transport immediately.

Gynecological Considerations

When dealing with any gynecological emergency outside of labor and delivery, never touch or insert your fingers or any object into the vagina. If there is bleeding, place a gauze pad on the outside of the vaginal opening to stem the bleeding. Keep track of any pain felt by the patient and, if the patient is bleeding, how much, but do not attempt any sort of physical exam. Monitor and manage other symptoms; keep any pads or gauze used as hemorrhage control to give to the hospital.

Chapter Summary

- The stages of labor and the signs of each one were identified along with the provider's role during each stage.
- The practice of delivery was covered, as to when to transport and how to support the patient during delivery.
- Possible complications that can occur during delivery were identified, as well as the change in procedure that needs to be considered for each complication.
- How to manage other gynecological emergencies and considerations in transport was covered.

Practice Questions
1. When should you consider delivering in the field instead of transporting a pregnant patient?

   (a) When a pregnant patient is asking you to
   (b) When contractions are 10 minutes apart
   (c) When you see crowning
   (d) When there are obvious birth complications

2. When, instead of crowning, you see the buttocks of the fetus, what type of delivery complication is it?

   (a) Limb presenting
   (b) Breech delivery
   (c) Placental abruption
   (d) Prolapsed cord

3. Once delivering a neonate in the field, you begin to assess them. You note that the babies' extremities are cyanotic, their heart rate is over 100 bpm, they have active movement and pull away from painful stimuli, and their respirations are slow and irregular. What would this baby's initial Apgar score be?

   (a) 6
   (b) 7
   (c) 8
   (d) 9

Chapter 15
Principles of Communications and Documenting

Introduction

At this point, you are already familiar that as a first responder, you work as part of a larger system. Thus, it is important to understand how to communicate properly with the other parts of the system—from dispatch and medical control to your partner who is right there in the truck with you. This also includes direct communication through your documentation of all aspects of the 911 call. Meticulous documentation is crucial for quality assurance and improved patient care.

Learning Objectives
Upon completing this section, you should be able to

- *understand* what information should be shared at each part of a call,
- *identify* what information should be shared at each part of a call,
- *infer* what method of communication would be appropriate at the time,
- *communicate* effectively and efficiently with others in EMS.

As we have previously learned, first responders have many different types of communication systems available to them, each with different levels of functionality. Each system uses frequencies which are regulated by the federal commission.

Base Station
These radio stations are stationary and are usually found at key locations such as dispatch buildings, hospitals, or other public safety facilities.

C. Ventura et al., *The Emergency Medical Responder*, https://doi.org/10.1007/978-3-030-64396-6_15

Mobile Two-Way Radios
These radios are also commonly known as transmitters and receivers and are mounted within a vehicle such as an ambulance, fire truck, or police cruiser. These radios are around 20–50 and not as strong as base stations. They can transmit a distance of 10–15 miles.

Portable Radios
These radios are handheld and have a power of around 1–5 watts and are thus limited in range.

Repeater Station
In order to increase efficiency and communication distance of the devices above, repeater stations are used. A repeater station is a stationary radio which will take in low-power signals and amplify them so they can be sent to a more distant location.

Cell Phones
That fancy piece of metal you keep in your pocket to text your friends, call your great grandmother who hasn't learned how to text yet, and play games when you're bored is occasionally used in EMS but is not a secure line for transmission of patient information.

It is critical that these methods of communication function and receive regular service as they are critical to the functioning of the EMS system. These are the currently available systems. But as time goes on, these systems will continue to improve.

When communicating via radio, there are some things that most people would consider common sense but are often forgotten. Firstly, push the "push to talk" button, and wait for 1 second before talking. Additionally, hold the microphone 2–3 inches from your face.

Considerations for Radio Communications
- Address the unit being called, and then, state the unit the call is coming from, and the receiving unit will let you know if they are available to talk by saying "go ahead" or "stand by."
- When finished with a communication, say "over," and get confirmation that it was received.
- You should minimize communication time by stating only the important information while avoiding special codes or excess phrases.
- Radio frequencies are not always secure; thus, patient personally identification information should not be used via radio.
- Ensure words are not mistaken and clear by saying the number followed by the individual digits and using affirmative and negative instead of yes and no.

Times to Notify Dispatch
You should notify dispatch when

- the call is received,
- en route to location,
- you arrive on location,
- you are at the patient,
- you are en route to the receiving facility,
- you are returning to base,
- you are back at base and clear.

What to Give in a Radio Report (Hospital Patch)
- Your unit and your provider level (EMR, EMT, paramedic).
- The age and sex of the patient.
- Chief complaint.
- Mechanism of injury or nature of illness.
- Past pertinent medical history.
- Mental status of the patient.
- Assessment findings and vital signs.
- What you have done to care for the patient.
- Estimated time to receiving facility.
- Ask if there are any remaining questions.

When you arrive at the hospital, you will need to give your report to the receiving staff. When you do this, you are essentially going to give them a shortened version of the radio report which is to include the patient's name, chief complaint, history, vital signs, treatments, and any additional information not given previously via radio.

Remember that radio communication can be confusing and things can be misheard. If there is ever any confusion and any situation you cannot hear properly or you hear something you think sounds unusual, don't be afraid to ask for a repeat or clarification.

Charting is one of the tasks that has made its way into the medical fields more and more over the years in hospitals, clinics, and even EMS. You may find out that charting is not necessarily the most exciting part of an EMS and dread doing it, but still it is of great importance. Yes, charts are necessary for insurance and billing purposes, but the reason why it is important is because it allows for a greater continuity of care for the patient. It allows other medical professionals to use that information to come up with a diagnosis and what treatment is indicated. The chart is also a legal document which can be used in court. Also, note that charts can be used for educational purposes to teach others as well as improve EMS systems. For these reasons, it is important that your charts are clear and accurate.

When running a call, there are pieces of information that you should consider and note which will be important for your report to the hospital as well as the chart. This is called the minimum data set. There may be variances in how charting is done at your specific agency, such as if it's digital or paper charts, but you must include the minimum data set.

Minimum Data Set
- Chief complaint
- Level of consciousness
- Mental status of the patient
- Systolic blood pressure
- Skin color, temperature, and condition
- Pulse rate
- Respiratory rate and effort
- Time (all the times dispatch was notified, e.g., en route, at patient, at receiving facility)

If you catch yourself making an error while charting, you must put a single line through the error, initial above it, and then write the correction after it. If you catch it after the chart is submitted, you should put a single line through the error, initially above it, but in a different color ink and add a note with the corrected information. If you just omitted information, you can simply add a note with your initials, the date, and the missing information.

When a patient refuses care, you must still write a patient care report on that call. In this type of chart, you will want to first explain to the patient that you recommend treatment and the risks that come with refusal. If the patient still refuses care, have them sign a refusal of care form. Additionally, have a witness such as a police officer, family member, or bystander sign saying that the patient refused care. In your patient care report, include any information you do have, such as anything you saw or noticed along, with what you would have wanted to do in terms of assessment and treatment.

If there are any special circumstances such as mechanical issues, ambulance crash, or personal injury, you can report that in a special report. Again, these are just general guidelines. Always refer to your agency and state protocols for documenting and reporting specifics. When writing your chart, try to maintain complete accuracy and clarity even if you make an error in your care. Document the error and write how you attempted to resolve it. The following sample patient care reports are examples not based on any real events.

Sample Patient Care Report No. 1

Arrived on scene to a 14-year-old M supine—legs elevated, A/AVPU, and GCS: 15. EMT Van Court took immediate C-spine immobilization, while EMT Denton documented pt's hx from parents. A spinal assessment was performed and a C-collar was applied. Pt reported of posterior neck pain with point tenderness and pain reproducible upon palpation after falling from a tree approx. 45 feet. Full neck range of motion restricted. A transport decision was made based upon agency trauma protocol. Pt was log rolled onto a backboard and was lifted to the stretcher. Pt was unremarkably loaded into the ambulance. No belongings transported. A head, neck, and spinal assessment was performed, and venous access was established at the right AC. A cold pack was applied to the superior head/parietal region with acute relief. CMS was assessed before and after each time pt was moved and once at the receiving facility. Normal distal and circulatory function in all extremities at all times of assessment. Upon arrival, pt was transferred to hospital stretcher via five-person lift. Hand-off report was given to RN, and pt's mother signed consent to tx form. Standard decontamination practices of stretcher and pt compartment were observed. Back in service 08:54.

C (chief complaint): Back/neck pain.

H (history): Dispatched to a residential area/home for a 14-year-old male, weight approx. 56 kg, and complaining of traumatic injury from fall.

A (assessment): Mental status: normal baseline for patient; neuro: normal baseline for patient; head: swelling, tenderness, and pain; face: normal; neck: pain and tenderness; chest/lungs: normal, left, and normal, right.

Rx (rendered treatment): Procedure: advanced spinal assessment x one successful; procedure: assessment, child x one successful; procedure: assessment, child x one successful; procedure: spinal motion restriction x one successful; procedure: application of cervical collar x one successful; procedure: venous access peripheral (IV) x one successful; and procedure: cold pack x one successful.

T (transport): The patient was transported emergent (immediate response), lights and sirens.

D (destination): The patient was transported to University Hospital 2. The destination was determined by agency trauma protocol.

Alena K.

EMT

#55555

Sample Patient Care Report No. 2

Arrived on scene with PD to a 74-year-old F: V/AVPU, GCS: 14, and A&OX2—disoriented to location and situation. CC: altered mental status. Husband reports pt woke from sleep to go to the bathroom and then did not want to return to bed. Pt became verbally combative toward husband, and 911 was called. EMT Ventura obtained a set of vital signs in the dining room. Pt was initially non-transport as per husband's preference; however, pt began to become verbally combative and disoriented again, so a transport decision to University Hospital 1 was made via family choice. PD cleared from scene.

Pt was walk-assisted by EMT Denton and EMT Ventura (as per preference) from the house to the ambulance, and the pt entered through the side door and was able to seat himself unremarkably. En route to the hospital, pt was cooperative and noncombative at all times of assessment and transport. A 12-lead was acquired, noting sinus bradycardia with second-degree AV block type II along with three sets of vitals during transport. Two unsuccessful BGL stick attempts were made. Pt was an unreliable historian and was unable to relay any medical hx. Pt provided an incorrect DOB, address, and middle name when asked. A list of medications was provided by the husband. Remaining transport time was uneventful, and signature for consent to tx was unobtainable from the pt. Upon arrival at the hospital, pt was moved via five-person lift over to hospital stretcher. Hand-off report was given to RN, and RN signed off in place of pt due to pt's mental status. Standard decontamination practices of stretcher and pt compartment were observed. Back in service with no delay.

R. Doe
NREMT
654,321

Sample Patient Care Report No. 3

C (chief complaint): R hip and back; knee pain.

H (history): Dispatched to a private residence/home for a 34-year-old female, weight approx. 92 kg, and complaining of back pain (nontraumatic). When obtaining pt history, she told us that he began experiencing pain in his back about 1.5 weeks ago and began seeing her chiropractor. She saw her orthopedic physician earlier today at Mercy, who is suspicious of a disc issue and was supposed to be getting an MRI. It began hurting more this evening, and his wife helped him with his Toradol around 18:00. He ate dinner of hamburger, pasta salad, and squash around 19:00. When 911 was called, he said his pain was a 10/10.

A (assessment): 21:20 mental status: normal baseline for patient, neuro: normal baseline for patient, head: normal, and face: normal. When Ed Coburn and I arrived on scene, we were met by Chase Ackerman and Christian Ventura, who had already assessed the patient. The patient was moved outside by a stair chair.

Once outside, he was transferred to the stretcher and then into the ambulance.

Patient's wife tried taking him by pov, but when the patient was standing, he began to pass out, and his wife could not hold him up, and the patient was not able to get into a position of comfort for transport by pov.

Rx (rendered treatment): Routine patient care, complete set of vitals, and patient comfort.

T (transport): The patient was transported emergent (immediate response).

Ride to GMC was uneventful. Pt care was transferred to ED nurse on duty in room no. 3.

D (destination): The patient was transported to Gifford Medical Center.

The destination was determined by closest facility.

Signed,

EMT Murray

Medic 4

Sample Patient Care Report No. 4

D: Dolliver Medic 2 was dispatched for a 34-year-old male that had fallen.

C: Pt fell and was unsure of what caused the fall. Pt had a 4 cm cheek laceration and was missing two teeth with minimal bleeding.

H: Pt does not have a history of falls. Pt was prescribed a new BP medication recently. Pt reports showering prior to the fall and may have moved too quickly. PMHx of diabetes, HTN, high BP, and depression.

A: On arrival, Pt was in a semi-Fowler's position and leaned up against a wall. Bystanders report they saw the pt fall face first into concrete. "He may have passed out or tripped." Pt reports no head or neck pain, but a C-collar was placed for precautions. Pt reports feeling nauseous and dizzy.

En route, a 12-lead ECG was acquired and was unremarkable. BGL was 158. Pupils were equal and reactive to light. Normal circulatory and distal function in all extremities.

R: Pt was given a C-collar to prevent spinal motion. Vitals were monitored en route.

T: Pt was sitting on the ground after moving from falling. C-collar was applied, and pt was able to stand and pivot onto the stretcher. Pt was secured in a supine position with straps and was loaded into the ambulance unremarkably. Throughout transport, vitals were monitored and remained stable. Pt was moved on the ER bed with a five-person sheet lift.

Report was given to a nurse at university hospital ER. All signatures were obtained.

V. Fanarjian

EMR

Unit 2

Sample Call Type/Location/Disposition
Service requested:

- 911 response (scene)

  Disposition:

- Patient treated, transported by this EMS unit

  Dispatch call type:

- Fall(s)

  Transport mode:

- Emergent (immediate response)

  Resp. mode:

- Emergent (immediate response)

  Urgency:

- Immediate

  Destination:

- University Hospital
- 1 Springer Way
- Great Barrington, MA, 01230

  Dest. determ.:

- Closest facility

  Location:

- Private residence/home

  Response delay:

- None/no delay

  Transport delay:

- None/no delay

Tips and tricks for writing a good narrative:

- Write using passive voice: Say "Vital signs were obtained at…" **not** "I took vitals…."
- Use acronyms when appropriate and universally understood (such as GCS or AVPU).
- Write what you saw/heard/observed **not** what you think you observed—although you can say "Bystander reported that the pt…etc."
- Use 24 hour time.
- Use your units (mmHg, BPM, SPO2%, etc.)!
- Saying DCAP-BTLS is okay!
- Remember, falsifying any information is illegal—**never** lie.
- Check spelling and grammar, always.
- If there is a pertinent quote you need to include in your report, put the patient's words in quotation marks.
- Identify if the patient is a reliable historian with regard to their medical history and demographics. Your dementia patient may give you a wrong date of birth, and your 13-year-old patient might now know he has Wolff-Parkinson-White syndrome.
- For traumatic incidents, mechanism of injury is important. Paint a picture of what happened.
- If you did it, you need to write it.
- If you didn't write it in the narrative, it didn't happen.
- Treat a PCR/narrative as a legal document. It is. Assume you will need to defend your treatment plan to a judge, each and every time you write one.

Chapter Summary

- When communicating via radio, try to remain as concise as possible while conveying all necessary information in a clear manner. Clarify any information that is not heard or was potentially misunderstood.
- All findings and treatments within an EMS call should be documented accurately and clearly to support continuity of care and further system improvement.

Practice Questions

1. When should you **not** notify dispatch of your actions?

   (a) En route to location
   (b) When your team is receiving the call
   (c) When you have returned to the station
   (d) When you are assessing a patient

2. When a patient wants to refuse any further care, what do you document?

   (a) You don't need to file a report as no care was given.
   (b) You file a refusal of care form with no additional report.
   (c) You write a report indicating the refusal of care and pair it with a signed refusal of care form.
   (d) You call the patient's physician to file a report with them.

3. What is **not** a part of the minimum data set?

   (a) Systolic blood pressure
   (b) Chief complaint
   (c) Pulse rate
   (d) Secondary neurological exam

Chapter 16
EMS Operations

Introduction

The job of an EMS clinician is not all about practicing medicine and saving lives. The role also includes some additional work in other areas which are not as glamorous. These are designated under the area of EMS operations and allow for there to be smooth functioning of EMS from a larger system to the individual first responder. This chapter will include topics such as safety in high-danger situations, responding on highways, and how to extricate a patient from a vehicle.

Transport Operations

Learning Objectives
Upon completing this section, you should be able to

- *understand* what actions must be performed in each phase of a call,
- *identify* what phase of a call is occurring,
- *infer* when air transport is necessary,
- *communicate* a verbal report to the receiving facility.

If you ask a random person off the street what an EMT does, there is a fairly high probability that they will say they are ambulance drivers and that they just throw the patient into the back of the truck so they can be brought to the hospital. As you have hopefully learned so far, EMTs do a lot more. Part of the job is transporting the patient to a hospital to receive definitive care.

© The Author(s), under exclusive license to Springer Nature Switzerland AG 2021
C. Ventura et al., *The Emergency Medical Responder*,
https://doi.org/10.1007/978-3-030-64396-6_16

The first phase of an EMS call happens before anyone even calls 911. This is known as the preparation phase. The majority of this phase consists of a rig check. A rig check includes going over all medical equipment in the ambulance to make sure it is not only present but also fully functional, as well as ensuring all medications are suitable for use. You must also check the engine, gas levels, siren systems, and radio communications. Rig checks are typically done at least once a shift. It is important to note that an ambulance must be staffed with at least one driver and one provider at the EMT level at a minimum. It is also encouraged to review traffic and weather conditions beforehand to be able to arrive at a patient's location as quickly and safely as possible.

When a tone drops for an incoming call, this is known as the dispatch phase. It is a relatively brief phase, but proper actions can help you prepare for the following stages. Your heart may be racing, and you may feel a rush of adrenaline. You must remain calm and follow proper protocols.

Dispatchers are highly trained professionals who initially pick up the 911 call and connect the caller to the appropriate resource. Dispatchers are trained to collect key information from the caller, direct the caller to perform CPR if necessary, and send the appropriate resources such as fire, police, EMS, or any combination of the three. Dispatch will also be the ones who will send you additional resources when you request them. Dispatch may contact you in various ways, from the traditional radio communication to a notification via an app.

When dispatched to a call, it is critical that you respond quickly to each patient as fast as possible. When you receive a call from dispatch, they will be giving you critical information about the call which will allow you to prepare. This information will typically include age, gender, location, and a brief description of the complaint if available. It is important to note that there may be times all you get is a location and an unknown medical emergency.

You are now in the ambulance and driving to the patient. This is known as the en route phase of a call. This time can be taken to come up with a game plan for when you arrive such as who will do what and what equipment you may want to get out first. On the other hand, if you are the driver, you must also focus and arrive at the patient not only quickly but also safely. Keep in mind if lights and sirens will be used, and note for changes in weather conditions. It may be appropriate to request an escort if the scene is dangerous or unfamiliar. Drivers will typically undergo an emergency vehicle operator course, but driver requirements vary by state as well as individual agencies.

You finally arrive at the patient's location. This is called the arrival phase. Before you even turn off the ambulance, you must consider where to park the ambulance taking into account the scene. For example, you must park uphill from any hazardous materials spills or 100 ft. from a motor vehicle collision. You may also want to park the ambulance in a manner that protects you from incoming traffic. At this point, you should don all appropriate PPE. This not only includes standard infectious disease precautions but also environmental hazards such as wearing a reflective vest when working in the street or a traffic area. Consider if there are any hazards such as a chemical spill. In this case, you will want to look for a placard and determine if the scene is safe by using the Hazardous Materials Emergency Response

Guidebook. At this point, you will also request any additional resources to manage the hazardous material. Once the scene is determined to be safe, you can now assess, treat, and prepare the patient for transport.

Once the patient is secured and loaded into the ambulance, the transport phase can begin. In this phase, you will continue to provide ongoing care for the patient. You will also want to alert the receiving facility of your arrival, especially in the case of a critical patient such as a major trauma or a stroke so they can prepare. You may also need to complete prehospital "patch" radio reports prior to your arrival at the receiving facility.

Once you arrive at the receiving facility, you have reached the nicely named phase, *arrival at the receiving facility*. When you arrive, you will transfer care of the patient to another medical professional, typically a nurse. You will begin with a thorough verbal report including patient identification information, treatments given, and major assessment findings.

Once you have transferred care of the patient, you have entered the final stage, the post-run stage. In this stage, you will debrief the call and complete any remaining documentation or charting. You will also need to decontaminate the ambulance. This may include use of cleaning wipes or even a full ultraviolet light decontamination for infectious disease patients. It is also important to restock any medical supplies or medication used in the previous call. Throughout all phases in the call, it is important to inform dispatch of your progress.

As a BLS provider, you will typically be working on a ground transport unit, but there will be times when air transport via a fixed wing or rotary wing may be used. When responding to a call, you may want to request air transport if transport time via ground is too long or if the patient is especially critical. When requesting air transport, keep in mind proper landing conditions are 100 ft. x 100 ft. of leveled clear ground. You will also want to report any possible hazards to dispatch. When the air ambulance arrives, the preferable approach is from the front of the helicopter, but a side approach may be used. You must never approach the helicopter from the rear. Fixed-wing air transport is typically used only for noncritical transport or long-distance transport. In this case, the plane will land at an airfield, and the ground unit will approach after the plane has come to a stop. In this case, you will be directed by airfield staff how and when to approach the plane.

Obtaining and Securing Access

Learning Objectives
Upon completing this section, you should be able to

- *understand* how and when to extract a patient in a safe manner,
- *identify* possible environmental dangers when responding to a call,
- *infer* risks of responding to traffic and highway incidents,
- *communicate* with other supporting resources for help when necessary.

Not all patients will be lying on the ground at a park or in their bed at home. You may come across a patient who is trapped in their car, on fire, and on the edge of a cliff. What do you do then? Of course, rule number one of EMS response is that your safety is the priority, then the other responders, and then finally your patient—because you can't help the patient if you become a patient. If there is any indication of danger, be sure to request the appropriate resources.

After the completion of an EMT program, you are only certified to extract a patient in limited scenarios, and there will be times when you are not trained to the level required to extract the patient. In addition to the EMT certification, you can ascertain training in extraction depending on the service you are working for, such as if you work for a fire department or rescue squad.

When considering extraction, your priority should be to treat the patient as much as you can before extraction to mitigate the damage that can occur from extraction. There is a case when extraction may occur first, and this is when you are unable to provide necessary care because of the current position or location of the patient. If an unstable patient is unable to be transported to a hospital, you should request an ALS unit or even an EMS physician unit if available. It is also important to determine which type of access you have. The two types of extrication include simple and complex access. The determining factor of which type of access you have is if special equipment, such as the jaws of life, are required. If the answer is yes, you do need special tools; it is complex access. If the answer is no, it is simple access.

You should also look for possible hazards before approaching the patient, such as downed power lines or fires. In the event there are downed power lines, maintain a safe distance, and notify dispatch that the power line must be turned off prior to safe patient care. This is especially true in a wet environment. In the event of a fire, you should request the fire department. You may also want to perform a rapid extraction if it is safe for you and your partner. If you are responding to an unstable vehicle, do not enter it and wait for additional resources.

When extracting the patient, it is important to protect the patient from dangers. An example of this is directing the patient to cover themselves with a blanket to protect them from glass shards if you are going to break the window. Additionally, consider spinal stabilization with equipment such as a KED, cervical collar, and a short or long backboard. Keep in mind that there will be scenarios when there is not enough time for full spinal stabilization and a rapid extraction must be used such as in the case of a fire. In most cases, it is acceptable for a patient to self-extricate themselves so long as a cervical collar is in place and no other gross deformities exist.

Chapter Summary

- Each EMS call will have similar phases such as en route, transport at facility, and leaving the facility, and each have items that must be addressed to provide efficient care.

- Air medical transport may be used in the case of a critical patient or if there is significant transport time to an appropriate receiving facility.
- Ensure your safety when responding to a patient. It is usually best to wait for extraction by qualified additional resources unless it puts the patient's life at risk.

Practice Questions

1. What is the first phase of any EMS call?

   (a) En route phase
   (b) Arrival phase
   (c) Preparation phase

2. What makes an extraction a simple access extraction instead of a complex access extraction?

   (a) A simple access extraction has only one patient involved.
   (b) A simple access extraction does not require special tools.
   (c) A simple access extraction has a wider opening to the patient.
   (d) A simple access extraction is only vehicular extraction.

3. What is the first step to approaching a patient for extraction?

   (a) Assessing what tools will be needed
   (b) Assessing whether the patient is stable or unstable
   (c) Assessing from where the patient needs to be extracted
   (d) Assessing the scene for any hazard to either you or the patient

Chapter 17
Well-Being of the First Responder

Introduction

EMS is an inherently stressful field with its hefty share of ups and downs. As a first responder, it is your duty to assure you are well cared for. You owe it to yourself, your colleagues, and your patients. This chapter will discuss healthy and unhealthy coping mechanisms, sources of on-the-job stress, and resources available to you.

> **Learning Objectives**
> Upon completing this section, you should be able to
>
> - *understand* sources of stress,
> - *identify* unhealthy coping mechanisms,
> - *infer* health methods for dealing with stress,
> - *communicate* with a friend when you need it!

In Chap. 12, we briefly touched on the process of grieving and methods to healthily progress through each step. As a first responder, you will inevitably come across stressful situations where you might need additional support, and that's okay! The EMS community continues to work incredibly hard to destigmatize the practice of asking for support. It's important to be able to get an idea of what events might impact your mental health and devise a plan for you to be able to get back on your feet.

Some examples of stressful events include exposure to the following:

- Loss of life, extremities, or organs
- Domestic, child, and elderly abuse
- Mass casualty/warm zone situations
- Encountering emergencies outside the scope of your training and/or confidence

© The Author(s), under exclusive license to Springer Nature
Switzerland AG 2021
C. Ventura et al., *The Emergency Medical Responder*,
https://doi.org/10.1007/978-3-030-64396-6_17

Stress can manifest in an infinite amount of ways, ranging from social to physical presentations. Some of these include the following:

- General anxiousness
- Difficulty concentrating
- Sleeping issues
- Irritability
- Loss of appetite/sexual arousal
- Decrease in work/social interactions

Healthy coping mechanisms should ideally be explored, with the understanding that seeking help is a tough task. First responders are encouraged to consider adjusting their lifestyle to support their overall health, by considering the following:

- Eating health, avoiding sugary, salty, and fatty foods whenever possible
- Engaging in at least 30 minutes of exercise every day
- Talking to a friend, family member, or clergy member
- Seeking support from a licensed social worker, clinician, therapist, or other mental health provider

Agencies are encouraged to consider implementing Critical Incident Stress Debriefing (CISD), which is a form of psychological therapy where mental health professionals coach personnel with processing their thoughts and feelings in a group setting or one-on-one. This typically occurs within 72 hours of the incident and is an incredibly effective tool for supporting the long-term health of all staff involved.

List of Available Resources Available to You! You Are Always Welcome to Use Them
Crisis Text Line:

- Text "EMS" to 741-741

  National Suicide Prevention Lifeline: For youth and adults:

- (800) 273-TALK (8255)

  American Association of Poison Control Centers:

- (800) 222-1222

  National Eating Disorders Center Helpline:

- (800) 931-2237
- Open M–F, 9–9 pm

  Veteran's Crisis Line:

- (800) 273-8255

YouthLine:

- (877) 968-8491
- Text TEEN2TEEN to 839-863

Rape, Sexual Assault, Abuse, and Incest National Network (RAINN):

- (800) 656-HOPE

National Domestic Violence Hotline/Child Abuse/Sexual Abuse:

- (800) 799-7233

SAMHSA's National Helpline:

- (800) 662-4357

National Institute on Drug Abuse Hotline:

- (800) 662-4357

EMS providers are encouraged and expected to take prophylactic precautions for their own health and well-being. This includes the use of body substance isolation (BSI) precautions, personal protective equipment (PPE), and required immunizations and testing (such as tetanus, hepatitis B, and tuberculosis testing).

Standard PPE typically includes the following:

- Non-latex gloves
- Surgical mask
- Goggles or face shield

Extra PPE may be worn in specific hazardous conditions. The "Emergency Response Handbook" and placards are helpful tools for identifying potential hazards. Remember that EMS providers can only provide life-sustaining care when it is safe to do so!

Chapter 18
Pandemic Response

Introduction

This chapter will discuss the role of emergency medical services in a pandemic with consideration of recent breakthrough science arising from the COVID-19 global emergency. Data and science included in this chapter are up to date at time of publication.

Learning Objectives
Upon completing this section, you should be able to

- *understand* the vectors of disease propagation,
- *identify* different levels of outbreaks,
- *infer* best practices for disease transmission mitigation,
- *communicate* the need for continued scientific investigation.

In the late months of 2019, pneumonia-like symptoms began to flood and intimidate families in Wuhan, China, which ignited a historic foreshadow of what would soon follow. It was not long before Chinese officials alerted the World Health Organization, and hurried investigation into this concerning symptomatology was commenced—for a virus which would later be named *severe acute respiratory syndrome coronavirus 2 (SARS-CoV-2)*.

Coronavirus disease 2019 (COVID-19) took the world by a storm and quickly exceeded the healthcare system capacity at almost every level in almost every country. ICU beds were at max capacity, ventilators were running out, and PPE ranged from hand-sewed cloth masks to artisanally repurposed vacuum cleaner bags. Evidently, our medical first responders took one of the hardest hits in the United States—overwhelming already short-staffed ambulance agencies, revisiting decontamination practices, and evaluating how providers would come back home safely to their families without exposing them to unnecessary risk.

In March 2020, the Health Advocacy and Medical Exploration Society (HAMES National) founded the Pro Bono EMS Pandemic Response Research Lab which aimed to investigate 911 and transport service response to COVID-19 using molecular biological, epidemiological, and anthropological methods. A national survey of EMS providers across the United States found that i) regular decontamination of EMS patient compartments and sanitation of personal stethoscopes are not common practices, ii) social distancing policies are not enforced by most EMS agencies, and iii) the majority of EMS providers report receiving no benefits related to COVID-19 response (Ventura et al. 2020). Researchers also found that despite the release of the CDC's Interim Guidance for EMS, many agencies and their providers felt lost and had implemented agency-specific approaches that were experimental or the staff's "best guess." Some state EMS offices began to encourage limiting the use of aerosolized procedures such as nebulizer treatments and rapid sequence intubation to decrease the likelihood of transmission of viral particles. Other states allowed agencies to devise their own approach to COVID-19 suspected cases. The following figure shows the official prehospital recommendations for responding to COVID-19 by the EMS Pandemic Response Research Lab.

In epidemiology, population analysis is a practice well visited by public health officials for understanding the severity of outbreaks. A situation can be classified as an *outbreak* when there is an unusually large amount of cases given the context of the environment and population. For example, in a college residential dorm facility of 500 students, eight cases of influenza would **not** be considered an outbreak. On the other hand, 250 cases of influenza would likely constitute an outbreak. To that end, one case of smallpox in a town of 1000 people would most certainly be considered an outbreak. An *epidemic*, however, occurs when an infectious disease becomes evidently contagious enough across a large geographical area. A *pandemic* is an epidemic that spreads across multiple large geographical areas, such as countries.

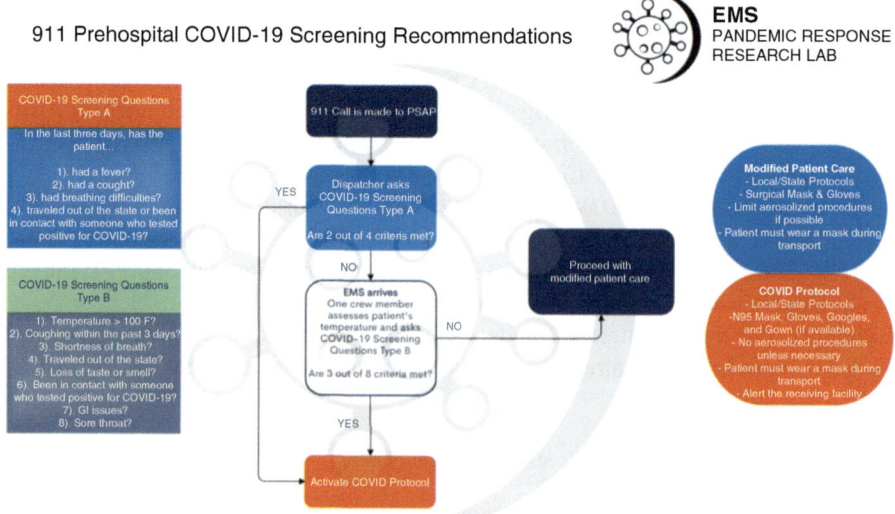

It is important to consider the three vectors of infectious disease transmission:

1. *Host*: Does the disease only infect humans, or animals too? What age range is mostly affected? Do these patients have other preexisting conditions?
2. *Pathogen*: What is the pathogen that is infectious? Is it a bacteria, virus, etc.? Could bioterrorism be involved?
3. *Environment/culture*: What factors in the environment are assisting in disease propagation? Is the disease spreading in a college dorm facility or in a nursing home? Are there cultural traditions that are affecting how the disease is transmitted from host to host?

To contain an outbreak, public health officials may institute/recommend a combination of the following disease mitigation practices: (This is not an extensive list.)

- *Social distancing*: Providing a 6 feet distance in between each person to avoid the transmission and receipt of respiratory droplets.
- *Face covering requirements*: Requiring people to wear a covering, such as a face mask, to decrease droplet transmission from the nose and mouth.
- *Quarantine*: Separating people from others for a specified time to see if they become sick.
- *Isolation*: Separating sick people from others who are not sick.
- *Cordon sanitaire*: Restricting people from entering and/or exiting a specified geographical region.

These public health precautions primarily assist in "flattening the epidemic curve" or slowing down disease transmission so as to not overwhelm the healthcare system capacity. Provider access to PPE, public health recommendation compliance, and continued public education are prerequisite to tackling outbreaks.

Chapter 19
Taking the NREMT Exam

The National Registry of Emergency Medical Technicians (NREMT) is a nonprofit organization based in Columbus, Ohio, that the majority of US states rely on to certify entry-level professional competency of EMS providers. The NREMT certifies emergency medical responders (NREMRs), basic emergency medical technicians (NREMTs), advanced EMTs (NRAEMTs), and paramedics (NRPs). While certification from the NREMT is not a license to practice, it is often the first step in obtaining state licensure.

NREMT-certified providers are "nationally registered" and must undergo two forms of testing—a cognitive written exam and a practical psychomotor exam. Applicants who successfully pass both assessments receive a card, patch, and certificate attesting to a provider's entry-level competency consistent with national EMS education standards. Some states accept the NREMT credential for direct reciprocity for state licensure, while other states may require passing of an additional psychomotor or cognitive exam. Most commonly, some states accept the NREMT credential in addition to a state EMS protocol in-service training.

> **The NREMT Cognitive Exam**
> "The National Registry Emergency Medical Technician (EMT) cognitive exam is a computer adaptive test (CAT). The number of items a candidate can expect on the EMT exam will range from 70 to 120. Each exam will have between 60 to 110 'live' items that count toward the final score. The exam will also have 10 pilot questions that do not affect the final score. The maximum amount of time given to complete the exam is 2 hours.

C. Ventura et al., *The Emergency Medical Responder*,
https://doi.org/10.1007/978-3-030-64396-6_19

The exam will cover the entire spectrum of EMS care including: Airway, Respiration & Ventilation; Cardiology & Resuscitation; Trauma; Medical; Obstetrics/Gynecology; EMS Operations. Items related to patient care are focused on adult and geriatric patients (85%) and pediatric patients (15%). In order to pass the exam, candidates must meet a standard level of competency. The passing standard is defined by the ability to provide safe and effective entry level emergency medical care."

Content area	Percent of exam	Adult/pediatric mix
Airway, respiratory, and ventilation	18–22%	85% adult; 15% pediatric
Cardiology and resuscitation	20–24%	85% adult; 15% pediatric
Trauma	14–18%	85% adult; 15% pediatric
Medical; obstetrics and gynecology	27–31%	85% adult; 15% pediatric
EMS operations	10–14%	N/A

Adapted from NREMT.org

The NREMT Cognitive Exam
"The National Registry Emergency Medical Responder (EMR) cognitive exam is a computer adaptive test (CAT). The number of items a candidate can expect on the EMR exam will range from 90 to 110. Each exam will have between 60 to 80 'live' items that count toward the final score. The exam will also have 30 pilot questions that do not affect the final score. The maximum amount of time given to complete the exam is 1 hour and 45 minutes.

The exam will cover the entire spectrum of EMS care including: Airway, Respiration & Ventilation; Cardiology & Resuscitation; Trauma; Medical; Obstetrics/Gynecology; EMS Operations. Items related to patient care are focused on adult and geriatric patients (85%) and pediatric patients (15%). In order to pass the exam, candidates must meet a standard level of competency. The passing standard is defined by the ability to provide safe and effective entry level emergency medical care."

Content area	Percent of exam	Adult/pediatric mix
Airway, respiratory, and ventilation	18–22%	85% adult; 15% pediatric
Cardiology and Resuscitation	20–24%	85% adult; 15% pediatric
Trauma	15–19%	85% adult; 15% pediatric
Medical; obstetrics and gynecology	27–31%	85% adult; 15% pediatric
EMS operations	11–15%	N/A

Adapted from NREMT.org

The psychomotor portion of the exam is handled through the state EMS office, although sometimes instructors are authorized to conduct psychomotor testing as part of the training program. See Chaps. 9 and 10 for help with the medical and trauma psychomotor assessment. Once you think you're ready, try completing the full-length practice exam in Chap. 20.

Luckily, the authors of this book have all taken the exam, and we're more than happy to share with you this exclusive list of tips and tricks:

1. Memorize and understand key vocabulary words; this can help you identify context clues if you don't fully understand the question.
2. Remember your priorities in this order: BSI, scene size-up, and ABCs.
3. To that note, you'll be surprised how much emphasis there may be on airway management. Think: hypoglycemic patients, head injuries, etc. Don't over-look this.
4. Look out for questions asking you what your *first* or *immediate* intervention is. This is **not** asking you about your overall treatment plan, but what you would do **first**.
5. Sometimes, there may be multiple right answers. Choose the **best** answer.
6. Sometimes, all the answers might be wrong. Choose the less wrong answer.
7. You might come across a question that appears as if there is not enough infor-mation. Choose the **best** answer and move on.
8. You get one question at a time, and you can't go back. Once you answer a ques-tion, forget about it, clear your mind, and move on to the next.
9. The exam is adaptive, meaning it's designed to make you feel like it's getting progressively more difficult. Take a deep breath; you got this!
10. If you realize you're spending lots of time on one question, guess and move on. There is no penalty for guessing. Process of elimination statistically gets you closer to the correct answer.
11. Try to take your exam early and on a weekday if you can. This is usually the quickest way to get your results back. Taking the exam on a weekend or Friday afternoon will require you to painfully wait longer for results.
12. There is no real way to find out if you passed until you receive your results on the NREMT website. The myths about having close to 70 questions or close to 100 are simply myths.

Chapter 20
Full-Length Practice Exam

Before You Begin
- Take a deep breath; you got this!
- Write your answers on a sheet of paper.
- Time yourself; aim to finish before 1.5 hours.
- Go in order; once you answer a question, you can't go back. This will prepare you for the real exam.
- Use the score analysis tool at the end of the exam to see our study recommendations.

1. A traumatic brain injury would be best described as:

   (a) Abnormal neurological symptoms associated with direct or indirect force to the brain
   (b) Focal neurological deficits as a result of a motor vehicle crash (MVC)
   (c) Unresolvable intracranial hemorrhaging that requires neurosurgical intervention
   (d) Light impact to the skull that leaves minor abrasions or contusions

2. Complete the sentence: The patient has an obvious left open radius fracture _____ to the shoulder.

   (a) Anterior
   (b) Proximal
   (c) Contralateral
   (d) Distal

C. Ventura et al., *The Emergency Medical Responder*, https://doi.org/10.1007/978-3-030-64396-6_20

3. Nystagmus is best defined as:

    (a) Nausea associated with vestibular eye movements
    (b) Rapid involuntary eye movements
    (c) Decrease in heart rate as a result of an oculocardiac reflex
    (d) Sensitivity to light

4. Which phase of a seizure is characterized by alternating contraction and relaxation of muscles?

    (a) Aura
    (b) Tonic
    (c) Clonic
    (d) Postictal

5. You arrive at the scene of a 6-year-old male patient who appears to be conscious and awake, but does not respond when you call his name. His eyes remain fixated, and his respirations are abnormally slow. The patient is most likely experiencing:

    (a) Complex partial (petit mal)
    (b) Cerebrovascular accident
    (c) Grand mal seizure
    (d) Febrile seizure

6. You arrive on scene to a 35-year-old male patient who presents with diaphoresis and a heart rate of 126 BPM. Which of the following is true?

    (a) The patient is cyanotic.
    (b) The patient is experiencing a complex partial seizure.
    (c) The patient is tachycardic.
    (d) The patient is bradycardic.

7. Which of the following is **not** a sign/symptom of congestive heart failure (CHF)?

    (a) Jugular venous distention
    (b) Pedal edema
    (c) Deviated trachea
    (d) Auscultated lung crackles

8. Which of the following is a contraindication of nitroglycerin (SL)?

    (a) Stable angina pectoris
    (b) Use of erectile dysfunction medication within the last 1–2 days
    (c) Hx of gastrointestinal bleeding in the last 2–3 months
    (d) All of the above

9. Which of the following is true?

    (a) Myocardial cells easily repair themselves.
    (b) Vasoconstriction increases arterial blood pressure.

(c) Vasodilation increases arterial blood pressure.

(d) 0.5 mg of renin-angiotensin IM is the treatment for NSTE-ACS.

10. Complete the sentence: Muffled heart sounds...

   (a) ...is always an indicator of cardiac compromise

   (b) ...when paired with jugular venous distention could indicate fluid in the pericardium

   (c) ...is never present in pediatric patients

   (d) Not enough information

11. You are treating a male patient with a GSW to the right posterior chest wall. Which of the following is an immediate concern?

   (a) Oximetry values should be obtained.

   (b) A blood pressure should be taken.

   (c) Apply direct pressure to the wound with a wet dressing.

   (d) An occlusive dressing should be applied along with checking for an exit wound.

12. Which combination of signs and symptoms could indicate the presence of a tension pneumothorax?

   (a) Bilateral wheezing and jugular venous distention

   (b) Absent lung sounds, deviated trachea, and obvious open chest wound

   (c) Rales at the base, tachypnea, and pedal edema

   (d) Not enough information

13. The treatment for acute anaphylaxis in a pediatric patient is:

   (a) 0.3 mg epinephrine (IM) 1:1000

   (b) 0.15 mg epinephrine (IM) 1:2000

   (c) 1 mg epinephrine (IV) q 3–5 min

   (d) 4 mg naloxone hydrochloride (IN)

14. Which of the following is true?

   (a) Oxygen therapy is always indicated in patients suspected of cardiac compromise.

   (b) A systolic of 142 mmHg is considered a hypertensive crisis.

   (c) Albuterol sulfate is the first drug consideration for patients in acute anaphylaxis.

   (d) Patients in a tripod position could indicate potential respiratory compromise.

15. Which of the following pair of signs and symptoms is the **best** indicator of respiratory arrest?

   (a) An SPO2 reading of 88% or lower

   (b) No breathing and no pulse

   (c) A faint radial pulse

   (d) No breathing with a palpable pulse

16. Which of the following is true?

    (a) As glucose rises, blood pressure decreases.
    (b) Hyperglycemia is associated with low insulin levels.
    (c) Blood sugar levels and insulin levels are directly proportional.
    (d) Beck's triad could indicate increased intracranial pressure.

17. Which of the following **does not** need to be considered before administration
    of oral glucose?

    (a) Verification of a positive gag reflex
    (b) The ability to follow commands
    (c) A systolic blood pressure < 90 mmHg
    (d) Not enough information

18. Which of the following might you find during the secondary assessment of a
    trauma assessment?

    (a) Secretions in the airway
    (b) A tachycardia heart rate
    (c) Decreased lung sounds over the left anterior thoracic wall
    (d) A major life threat like arterial hemorrhaging

19. During which part of a medical assessment would you identify any respiratory
    concerns?

    (a) Primary assessment
    (b) Secondary assessment
    (c) Tertiary assessment
    (d) OPQRST

20. Why is it important to reassess a patient regularly?

    (a) To check for anything you may have missed
    (b) To provide the patient with emotional support
    (c) To check for any changes in the patient's condition
    (d) Not enough information

21. You respond to a call for a 42-year-old woman with severe abdominal pain. The
    patient points to the lower left side of her abdomen. You report the region of the
    patient's pain as the:

    (a) LUQ
    (b) LLQ
    (c) RLQ
    (d) RUQ

22. A patient reports feeling lightheaded after fasting all day. This most likely
    affects which of the following body systems?

    (a) Circulatory system
    (b) Endocrine system

(c) Musculoskeletal system

(d) Nervous system

23. You are assessing a 15-year-old male patient who is febrile and complaining of pain in the RLQ region. Which condition is the patient most likely experiencing?

(a) Ectopic pregnancy

(b) Pancreatitis

(c) Appendicitis

(d) Chronic constipation

24. You respond to a call for a motorcyclist who was ejected. As you arrive, the patient is lying with her face toward the ground, on her abdomen. This is known as what type of position?

(a) Lateral

(b) Prone

(c) Semi-Fowler's

(d) Supine

25. Which of the following would be an expected response to parasympathetic stimulation?

(a) Heart rate decreases.

(b) Tachypnea.

(c) Smelling enhances.

(d) Tripod position.

26. Which of the following is the biological unit of energy used in humans?

(a) Cellulose

(b) Mitochondria

(c) RNA

(d) ATP

27. Which of the following heart rhythms is usually responsible for cardiac arrest?

(a) Tachycardia

(b) Ventricular fibrillation

(c) Sinus rhythm

(d) Bradypnea

28. You are responding to a 29-year-old female patient who was ejected from an automobile and is now unresponsive. You note unequal pupils which is indicative of bleeding in the brain. Which of the following combinations of blood pressure, respiratory rate, and heart rate is indicative of neurological compromise?

(a) BP: 156/92 mm/Hg, RR: 6/min, and HR: 40 BPM

(b) BP: 120/80 mm/Hg, RR: 12/min, and HR: 74 BPM

    (c) BP: 84/60 mm/Hg, RR: 88/min, and HR: 100 BPM

    (d) BP: 122/82 mm/Hg, RR: 14/min, and HR: 82 BPM

29. A patient who has a fluid-based airway obstruction would most likely present with:

    (a) Snoring

    (b) Gurgling

    (c) Wheezing

    (d) Rhonchi

30. The BLS primary assessment goes as follows:

    (a) BSI and scene size-up, check for responsiveness, check for breathing and pulse simultaneously, activate the emergency response system, and start CPR.

    (b) BSI and scene size-up, activate the emergency response system, check for breathing and pulse simultaneously, and start CPR.

    (c) BSI and scene size-up, check for responsiveness, activate the emergency response system, check for breathing and pulse simultaneously, and start CPR.

    (d) BSI and scene size-up, check for responsiveness, activate the emergency response system, check for breathing, check for pulse, and start CPR.

31. Human body cells replicate through a process known as:

    (a) Binary fission

    (b) Mitosis

    (c) Cellular respiration

    (d) Photosynthesis

32. Which form would you use to document refusal of care?

    (a) DNAR form

    (b) Insurance claim form

    (c) CPSS form

    (d) Against medical advice form

33. You are treating a 42-year-old patient in a restaurant who appears as if she is choking but is able to briefly talk in short sentences. There are no indications of poor perfusion. Which of these is your most appropriate action?

    (a) Provide ten black slaps.

    (b) Perform abdominal thrusts.

    (c) Remove the obstruction with your hand.

    (d) Encourage the patient to continue coughing.

34. What is the recommended oxygen delivery rate for a non-rebreather mask?

    (a) 2–6 LPM

    (b) 1–5 LPM

(c) 6–8 LPM

(d) 10–15 LPM

35. What is the recommended oxygen delivery rate for a nasal cannula?

(a) 2–6 LPM

(b) 1–5 LPM

(c) 6–8 LPM

(d) 10–15 LPM

36. You are responding to the scene of a gunshot wound victim. What is your immediate priority?

(a) Conduct a scene size-up.

(b) Conduct a focused primary assessment.

(c) Apply an occlusive dressing to the patient.

(d) Not enough information.

37. You are called to the home of a 68-year-old female patient who says she feels pressure in chest radiating to her back. This is known as the patient's:

(a) AVPU

(b) General impression

(c) Nature of illness

(d) Chief complaint

38. Which of the following would you likely find during your secondary assessment?

(a) Whether the scene is unsafe

(b) The patient's pertinent medical history

(c) Arterial bleeding

(d) Any immediate life-threatening problems

39. What is the purpose of a primary survey?

(a) To identify any immediate life threats

(b) To obtain a patient history

(c) To identify any fractures

(d) All of the above

40. You will most likely find patients experiencing respiratory distress in which position?

(a) AVPU position

(b) Recovery position

(c) Recumbent position

(d) Tripod position

41. A patient who is hypoglycemic might be mistaken for:

(a) Being intoxicated

(b) Suffering an acute MI

(c) Having an asthma attack

(d) Experiencing right ventricular heart failure

42. Which of the Cincinnati Prehospital Stroke Scale (CPSS) is evaluated when you ask a suspected stroke patient to raise both arms?

(a) Auditory retention

(b) Arm drift

(c) Memory

(d) Aphasia

43. What is the normal resting heart rate range for an adult patient?

(a) 50–80 BPM

(b) 60–100 BPM

(c) 50–100 BPM

(d) 60–120 BPM

44. Applying a tourniquet to a patient is most likely indicated in:

(a) Arterial bleeding

(b) Capillary bleeding

(c) Venous bleeding

(d) All types of bleeding

45. You arrive at the scene of a motor vehicle collision in which a vehicle struck a large telephone pole. Which is the best indicator of potential injury?

(a) Height of the telephone pole

(b) Circumference of the telephone pole

(c) Mass of the patient

(d) Speed of the vehicle

46. Which is the most common cause of upper airway obstruction in the trauma patient?

(a) Blood

(b) Gums

(c) Tongue

(d) Cerebrospinal fluid

47. You should first attempt to open the airway of a trauma patient using which maneuver?

(a) Head-tilt/chin-lift

(b) Scissor method

(c) Cricoid method

(d) Jaw thrust

48. You are currently assessing an 87-year-old patient that is currently taking a prescribed medication you have never heard of before. You are unsure whether

this drug may pose as a contraindication. Which type of medical control should you initiate?

(a) Online medical control
(b) Offline medical control
(c) Standing orders
(d) Not enough information

49. You arrive on scene to treat a 47-year-old female for a suspected cardiac event. You are asked to comfort the patient's partner who is obviously anxious, sweating, and breathing rapidly. Which type of autonomic nervous system do you suspect is most dominant in the patient's partner?

(a) Sympathetic
(b) Parasympathetic
(c) Peripheral
(d) Integumentary

50. Which of the following scenarios would most likely be the most immediately life-threatening to a patient?

(a) External hemorrhage from a scalp laceration
(b) Internal hemorrhage in the subdural space due to a fall
(c) A missing segment of the skull from a blunt weapon attack
(d) Damage to the lumbar spinal cord in a car collision

51. You are assessing a suspected stroke patient who is unable to produce coherent speech. Which lobe of the brain is most likely afflicted?

(a) Frontal
(b) Temporal
(c) Parietal
(d) Occipital

52. You arrive at the scene of a 57-year-old patient who is the victim of suspected domestic violence. Upon your thorough questioning, it becomes evident that the patient is aware of their location, but not their identity or the time of day. This patient is:

(a) A&OX1
(b) A&OX2
(c) A&OX3
(d) A&OX4

53. You are called to the scene of a patient who has been assaulted and stabbed in the spine with a knife. You stabilize the knife and provide immediate transport while managing airway, breathing, and circulation of the patient. Which type of spinal injury does this patient likely have?

(a) Compression injury
(b) Penetrating injury

    (c) Hyperextension injury

    (d) Distraction injury

54. You are called to respond to an unconscious male who has fallen from a two-story building. The patient is unresponsive and is currently in a prone position. It is suspected that a spinal injury may be present. Which method of spinal stabilization is **not** indicated at any point in this situation?

    (a) Kendrick Extrication Device

    (b) Long backboard

    (c) Cervical spine collar

    (d) Manual spinal stabilization

55. You are responding to a 34-year-old male patient with shortness of breath. He has a history of COPD emphysema, type 1 diabetes, and an allergy to penicillin. Upon auscultation, you noticed decreased lung sounds over the left side of his posterior thorax. What condition is this patient most likely experiencing?

    (a) Asthma attack

    (b) Anaphylaxis

    (c) Hemothorax

    (d) Pneumothorax

56. You are responding to an 18-year-old female patient with shortness of breath in a tripod position. She has a history of mild asthma. Which of the following should be your first immediate intervention?

    (a) Apply a cervical collar.

    (b) Assist the patient with her inhaler.

    (c) Ventilate the patient with a BVM, 1 breath every 5–6 seconds.

    (d) Apply a non-rebreather mask at 15 LPM.

57. You arrive at the scene of a 50-year-old male complaining of chest pain. While taking a patient history, the patient reports that the pain started while he was mowing the lawn but lessened gradually when he sat down to wait for the ambulance. What type of angina does this patient have?

    (a) Stable angina

    (b) Unstable angina

    (c) Vasospastic angina

    (d) Vasodilatory angina

58. An automated external defibrillator (AED) reanalyzes a cardiac rhythm every:

    (a) 2 minutes

    (b) 6 minutes

    (c) 30 compressions

    (d) After ROSC

59. You are treating an elderly male patient whom you suspect to be having a heart attack. You administer 325 mg of aspirin and identify that the patient has been prescribed nitroglycerin by his cardiologist. You note the following vital signs: HR: 106 BPM, RR: 14 RPM, BP: 116/p, and O2: 98%. What question might you want to ask your patient before administering nitroglycerin?

    (a) Do you take any high blood pressure medication?
    (b) Have you taken any erectile dysfunction medication in the past 48 hours?
    (c) Are you allergic to penicillin?
    (d) How many times have you administered nitroglycerin in your lifetime?

60. You are treating an adult male patient for a gunshot wound to the right anterior chest wall. Which of the following is your first immediate action?

    (a) Apply sterile gauze to the wound.
    (b) Listen to lung sounds.
    (c) Apply a gloved hand directly to the wound.
    (d) Apply an occlusive dressing.

61. You arrive on scene to a 35-year-old male patient complaining of pressure-like chest pain who appears anxious and diaphoretic. You note the following vital signs: A&OX2, BP: 88/70 mmHg, RR: 14/min, HR: 104 BPM, and T: 97.8 F. Which of the following does this likely indicate?

    (a) The patient requires pulse oximetry immediately.
    (b) The patient fulfills the criteria for congestive heart failure.
    (c) The patient's chest pain is likely anxiety-induced.
    (d) The patient is unstable.

62. You are responding to a 12-year-old female patient who was ejected from a motor vehicle, likely due to not wearing a seatbelt. In your secondary assessment, you note the following vital signs: P on the AVPU scale, BP: 64/p mmHg, RR: 0/min, HR: 120 BPM, and SPO2: 84%. Which of the following is true?

    (a) The patient requires oxygenation via a bag valve mask device, one breath every 10 seconds.
    (b) The patient's blood pressure is highly indicative of cerebral hemorrhaging.
    (c) The patient is tachycardic.
    (d) The patient is tachypneic.

63. You are transporting a patient with a suspected injury that presents with a waxing and waning level of consciousness. Which of the following is your most primary concern?

    (a) Conducting a regular neurological exam
    (b) Maintaining an open airway

(c) Arriving to the hospital quickly

(d) Assessing regular distal function

64. You are responding to the scene of a pediatric patient, when his parents begin to start yelling at you angrily. You should immediately:

(a) Raise your voice to neutralize the situation.

(b) Transport the child without the parents in the patient compartment.

(c) Contact social services.

(d) Notify law enforcement.

65. Type II diabetes is generally secondary to:

(a) Genetics and lifestyle

(b) Lifestyle only

(c) High cholesterol

(d) A high body mass index (BMI)

66. You are attempting to resuscitate an 89-year-old female when a family member presents a DNAR form. Another family member begs you to keep performing CPR. You should:

(a) Acknowledge the form and stop resuscitation.

(b) Verify the authenticity of the form by calling the family's physician.

(c) Continue resuscitation at the request of the family member.

(d) Verify the authenticity of the form by calling the family's attorney.

67. The main difference in the stages of respiratory compromise is:

(a) How open the airway is

(b) The presence of compensatory mechanisms

(c) The oxygen saturation value

(d) The patient's systolic blood pressure

68. The condition characterized by decreased lung elasticity and moderate to severe alveolar damage is:

(a) Emphysema

(b) Bronchitis

(c) Pulmonary embolism

(d) Pneumothorax

69. Delivery is imminent once the contraction interval time is:

(a) 10–15 minutes

(b) 7–8 minutes

(c) Less than 15 minutes

(d) Less than 2 minutes

70. When the placenta separates early from the uterus at around 25 weeks, this is known as:

(a) Gestation
(b) Placenta previa
(c) Placental abruption
(d) Primigravida

Practice Test Answer Key

1. A.
2. D.
3. B.
4. C.
5. A.
6. C.
7. C.
8. B.
9. B.
10. B.
11. D.
12. B.
13. A.
14. D.
15. D.
16. B.
17. C.
18. C.
19. A.
20. C.
21. B.
22. B.
23. C.
24. B.
25. A.
26. D.
27. B.
28. A.
29. B.
30. B.
31. B.
32. D.
33. D.

34. D.
35. A.
36. A.
37. D.
38. B.
39. A.
40. D.
41. A.
42. B.
43. B.
44. A.
45. D.
46. C.
47. D.
48. A.
49. A.
50. B.
51. B.
52. A.
53. B.
54. A.
55. D.
56. D.
57. A.
58. A.
59. B.
60. C.
61. D.
62. C.
63. B.
64. D.
65. A.
66. A.
67. B.
68. A.
69. D.
70. C.

No. of questions correct	Score + recommendation
62–70	Pass: nice! Spend 10% studying for the cognitive exam and 90% on psychomotor skills.
59–61	Pass: good job! Spend 30% studying for the cognitive exam and 70% on psychomotor skills.
55–58	Pass: you might need to touch up on a particular topic. We recommend you spend most of your time reviewing for the cognitive exam.
50–54	Pass: you might need to thoroughly review each topic. We recommend you spend most of your time reviewing for the cognitive exam.
Below 50	Fail: please reread chapters you are not fully confident in. We recommend you spend most of your time reviewing for the cognitive exam before considering psychomotor skills practice.

Chapter 21
Appendix: Weapons of Mass Destruction and Bioterrorism

Introduction

No country, state, or city is immune to acts of terrorism, and it is the responsibility of EMS to be able to quickly adapt to the rapidly changing situations. In order to properly assess and treat victims of a terrorist attack, we must first understand the effects of various weapon types on the human body. We will also learn how to identify the weapon type used based off of a patient's presentation, to ensure proper treatment is given.

Learning Objectives
Upon completing this section, you should be able to

- *understand* what constitutes terrorism or a terrorist attack,
- *identify* the different forms of weapons of mass destruction,
- *infer* how your patient care may change in the event of terrorism,
- *communicate* effectively with the incident command team.

The FBI defines terrorism as "violent, criminal acts committed by individuals and/or groups to further ideological goals stemming from influences such as those of a political, religious, social, racial, or environmental nature." Terrorism is typically categorized into two groups: domestic and international. International terrorism is committed by organized foreign terrorist groups or the government of another nation. An almost universally known example of an international terrorist attack are the attacks of 11 September 2002 on the World Trade Center. Domestic terrorism is committed by one or more individuals within the country. An example of this would be the Boston Marathon Bombings of 15 April 2013. Terrorist attacks are traditionally violent and are motivated by radical ideological beliefs.

© The Author(s), under exclusive license to Springer Nature
Switzerland AG 2021
C. Ventura et al., *The Emergency Medical Responder*,
https://doi.org/10.1007/978-3-030-64396-6_21

Weapons of mass destruction come in many different forms, but most can be placed into one of four categories: biological weapons, chemical weapons, radiological weapons, and explosive weapons.

Biological Weapons

Biological weapons use microorganism or animal-derived products as its primary method of inflicting damage. Examples of microorganisms used in biological weapons include viruses and bacteria. Because of the wide variety of organisms that exist, there is an incredible amount of biological weapons that can be manufactured. Biologicals can pose a great threat as it is often hard to distinguish between a biological weapon attack and a common disease outbreak. The CDC has established three categories for biological weapons, A, B, and C, based on their threat level.

Levels of biological weapons		
Category A	Highly contagious or easily spread High mortality rate	Ebola Smallpox Anthrax
Category B	Moderately contagious Moderate mortality rate	Ricin toxin Brucellosis Typhus fever
Category C	Emerging pathogens which have the potential to be engineered for use as a biological weapon	Nipah virus Hantavirus

It is important to consider how biologicals affect specific organ systems. Review the following chart for examples. Remember that your primary objective is continued management of the airway, breathing, and circulation regardless of the biological weapon type.

Examples of organ systems targeted by microorganisms	
Neurological	Botulism Shiga toxin
Respiratory	SARS-CoV Plague
Cardiovascular and hematological	Ebola Viral hemorrhagic fever
Skin related	Smallpox T-2 mycotoxin

Chemical Weapons

Chemical weapons use nonliving chemicals to inflict death or illness to humans. Chemical weapons are often much easier and faster to identify than biological weapons. Luckily, there are some chemical weapons that have antidotes available to BLS providers.

Organophosphate poison functions as a nerve agent. In this condition, acetylcholinesterase is blocked by the toxin, causing an overaccumulation of acetylcholine. This then causes an overstimulation of neurons, eventually leading to death if not treated. The signs and symptoms of organophosphate poisoning can be remembered by using the mnemonic SLUDGE. It is especially important to be able to identify organophosphate poisoning because the primary reversal agent is *atropine sulfate*, which can be administered by first responders via an auto-injector.

SLUDGE acronym for organophosphate poisoning:

- S: Salivation
- L: Lacrimation
- U: Urination
- D: Diarrhea
- G: Gastrointestinal discomfort
- E: Emesis

Another primary category of chemical weapons is vesicants. Vesicants are categorized by the formation of blisters. While external blisters are painful, vesicants are especially dangerous because they can form within the airway causing it to be occluded. Advanced airway intervention is often indicated at first sign of the formation of airway blisters. Vesicants can also compromise other systems, such as the immune system and gastrointestinal system. A common example of a vesicant is mustard gas.

The third type of chemical weapons is respiratory agents. These either can have an irritant effect on the airway or can be more severe and act as an asphyxiant. Respiratory irritants often have a low mortality rate but can cause respiratory distress or pulmonary edema. Examples of respiratory irritants include chlorine, ammonia, and phosgene. As previously mentioned, asphyxiants are much more dangerous as they inhibit oxygen intake and interfere with oxygen displacement and/or cellular respiration. Examples of asphyxiants include carbon monoxide and hydrogen sulfate. Treatment of these chemical weapons is primarily management of respiratory and airway compromise.

Radiological Weapons
Radiological devices are used quite often throughout the field of medicine, from the treatment of cancers to imaging methods such as X-rays and MRIs. Despite its great usefulness, high levels of radiation can be dangerous, as it affects DNA replication and can cause damage to genomic information. Radiological weapons can take a while to detect as it can act from a distance. Additionally, radiation damage does not typically present with symptoms until days or weeks later. There is unfortunately little a first responder can do in this situation. The best course of action is to alert hazmat and law enforcement so that the radiological weapon can be contained and disposed of.

Explosive Weapons

Explosive weapons are bombs or other explosive devices that inflict great damage to property and/or people. Explosives can often be quickly identified when detonated. As a medical first responder, your role will be to treat traumatic injuries. You should treat these patients as you would any other trauma patient, referring to the trauma assessment and management of ABCs. You should also consider that explosives may also be combined with radiological and/or biological toxins. These are commonly known as "dirty bombs."

Although there exists a diverse amount of weapons that have the potential to cause great harm, there are some elements of EMS operations that remain constant. The first is always scene safety and the use of appropriate body substance isolation. If the scene is not safe for the first responder, they should not enter the environment without the assistance of specialized resources. If you are required to enter the environment, ensure you have the appropriate personal protective equipment whether it be gloves, a respirator, or even a full biohazard suit. Remember to follow proper local guidelines and triage protocols in the event you are responding to an act of terror.

Chapter 22
Appendix: Introduction to Triage and the Incident Command System

Introduction

Throughout the book, we have spoken about how to manage and treat patients in a one-to-one interaction, where there is one patient per team of providers. However, this is not always the case. There are many times where you will respond to an incident which has injured more than one person, meaning that you will find yourself responsible for multiple patients at a time. Also, in these multiple-casualty incidents, you will find yourself having to work closely with more people than just your partner or crew on the ambulance. You will be working in larger teams depending on the scale of the incident in which you are one of the responders too. How many EMS providers were present to treat victims of Hurricane Katrina? How did they have their roles assigned, and how did they coordinate with other rescue personnel? This chapter will give you a clear path to follow in what would otherwise be chaotic and complicated situations.

Triage

Learning Objectives
Upon completing this section, you should be able to

- *understand* what defines a mass casualty incident,
- *identify* the meanings of the different patient tags,
- *infer* which color belongs to each patient,
- *communicate* your patient's status with other providers.

C. Ventura et al., *The Emergency Medical Responder*, https://doi.org/10.1007/978-3-030-64396-6_22

Imagine that you are a provider in a two-person ambulance crew and you respond to a car crash. Upon arrival on scene, you find out that there were six people involved in the crash and five of them were injured. Both you and your partner can each work on one patient, but which of the five patients needs care the most and receives priority? To determine this, you will need to use the START triage system.

Triage is assigning priority of care to patients before providers begin to treat them. It is most commonly utilized during mass casualty incidents where the number of patients exceeds the amount of immediately available resources.

The START triage system allows providers to group patients into four priority categories. Patients who are tagged red are the highest-priority patients, signaling the need for immediate care. The second priority group is tagged yellow, meaning that they need care but that care can be delayed. The third priority group is green, meaning that they have minor injuries and can wait until after all other patients are transported. The final category is probably the most difficult one for a provider to assign, it is the black category which indicates a patient who is dead or expectant.

In order to tag people into these four categories, there is an algorithm for providers to follow:

1. Walking up to the scene, take note of the patients that are ambulatory, meaning they are able to walk, as these patients are automatically tagged green, and you can then move on to the nonambulatory patients.
2. The first sign to check in each patient is their respirations. If they are not breathing at all, even after you position their airway, they are tagged black. If their respirations are over 30 respirations a minute or you had to position their airway to allow them to breath, they are tagged red.
3. Next, you have to check their circulation. If their capillary refill is over 2 seconds or you cannot feel a radial pulse, make sure to immediately control any bleeding, and then, tag that patient red.
4. Finally, check to see if the patient can follow simple commands. If they cannot, they are tagged red; if they can, they are tagged yellow.

Red (immediate)	Respirations >30 per minute or upon repositioning of airway Absent radial pulse or capillary refill >2 seconds Unable to follow simple commands
Yellow (delayed)	Nonambulatory
Green	Ambulatory
Black (expectant)	No respirations

Now that that algorithm is understood, let's give an example of a situation in which this algorithm can be applied. Say there was a building collapse and those in charge of search and rescue were able to extricate five patients. Two of those patients are able to walk, one with a broken wrist and the other with a concussion, so you automatically tag them green, despite the other injuries. Moving on to the next patient, you find them breathing, with proper circulation, and able to follow your command to tell you their name, so you tag them yellow. The next patient is not breathing, and after trying to reposition their airway, they are still not breathing, so you tag them black. The final patient is tachypneic and breathing well over 30 breaths per minute, so you tag them red. So the order you will then treat the patient is the red-tagged, tachypneic patient first and then the nonambulatory, yellow-tagged patient second, and then, you will move on to the green-tagged patients. Once all other patients are taken care of, you can reassess the black-tagged patient.

Incident Command System

Learning Objectives
Upon completing this section, you should be able to

- *understand* when the incident command system is used,
- *identify* the different sections within the leadership hierarchy,
- *infer* your role within the system,
- *communicate* using common language with other personnel.

Imagine that you were one of the first responders to the attack on the World Trade Center. You are suddenly faced with thousands of potential patients and limited resources. How are you supposed to know what to do and how to work with the firefighters on scene, the police officers controlling the crowd, and the other EMS providers from other agencies? In these types of situations, you find yourself thrust into a confusing web of resources, personnel, and communications; however, there is a system put in place so that people can work effectively in midst of these large-scale catastrophes.

Before starting any job in EMS, you, as a provider, will have to take a large amount of additional ICS training. ICS stands for the incident command system. When there is a critical incident or there is an incident which crosses jurisdictional boundaries, this system is meant to create a hierarchy of leadership and help foster interorganizational cooperation to aid efficient emergency response. This is a prerequisite for most jobs in emergency response, but is not covered by the EMS curriculum. However, understanding the basics of the ICS now will help you prepare for the training you will have to complete later on and give you an idea of the system that you will enter.

The incident command system is utilized for emergency response to critical incidents. This includes wildfires, structural fires, search and rescue operations, and spills of hazardous materials, just to name a few. These types of incidents involve firefighters, policemen, EMS providers, and any other specialty personnel. These are large operations that can become very complicated, as all of the different personnel involved have their own chain of command, their own orders, and different people that they answer too. ICS simplifies this so that emergency response can happen as efficiently as possible without time being spent on figuring out which people to answer to and who to share information with.

The first step in the process is to establish an *incident commander*, the person in charge of overseeing the scene and all operations affecting it. This position changes often as it usually goes to the person on scene with the most experience in that area, and every new group of people who come and the larger the incident gets, more people with more experience enter the pool for this position. For example, if the first people to arrive at structure fire were an EMT and a paramedic, the paramedic would become the temporary incident commander. If, then, the fire chief arrived on scene, the paramedic would brief the chief on the incident, and that position would be handed over.

Different operations under the incident command are then divided into four divisions. There is the *operations section*, which directs tactical operations and tactical resources. Next is the *planning section*, which essentially is in charge of paperwork, filing documentation of the incidents, resources used, and personnel. After that, there is the *logistics section* which provides and sends out resources to those at the incident. Finally, there is the *finance and administration section*, which provides accounting and money management for the duration of the incident. It is in the creation of these sections where the flexibility of ICS shows, as not all of these divisions need to be created. Sometimes, in a small incident with a short operational period or timeframe in which the incident is responded to, the incident commander can fill the roles of all five sections without additional personnel. However, the larger the incident, the more sections are needed for proper incident management. The larger the incident, the more a chain of command is also important, as the ICS standard is that for every supervisor, there are no more than five personnel. This flexibility in the face of differing scales and events is why the incident command system was created, along with the clear route of communication it provides.

Along with a divided organizational structure, there are specific leadership positions which run each section and aid the incident commander. Besides the incident commander, three other people hold leadership roles within the incident command, making up the command staff. The first is the safety officer, who oversees the safety precautions being taken for both the providers and the patients at the incident. Second is the liaison officer who serves as the point of contact between the incident command and all supporting agencies and divisions. Third is the public information officer who is the point of contact for news organizations, the media, and the larger public. Under the command staff, each of the previously mentioned sections has a section chief presiding over them.

Besides understanding the structure of the ICS leadership, you will also need to know the purpose of different locations that will be set up for the purpose of incident management. There will be a location designated for the incident command staff called the incident command post. Most of the incident oversight will occur from this location. The base is where the majority of support operations and services are organized. Staging areas and camps are where resources are held and prepared for distribution.

This makes up the basic structure of the incident command system, but now, you need to know how it will apply to your position on scene. While working on scene, you will be briefed and overseen by a direct supervisor as a part of one of the sections. As you are an EMS provider, you will most likely fall under the operations section. It is important to understand the role given to you by your supervisor in order to do your job effectively. It is also important to understand all of the terminology used throughout this chapter so that you can effectively communicate with whoever you come into contact with. The usage of common language as described by all of the ICS training that you will receive will make sure that your actions and the briefing given to you are understood by all relevant personnel.

Chapter 23
Appendix: Patient Extrication

Introduction

Even though most people envision the scene of a medical emergency to be that they just happen to collapse on the sidewalk where they can easily be loaded into the back of the ambulance, this is very rarely the case. It is more common that the patient will be in a car or on a hiking trail, and as an EMT, it is your responsibility that the patient receives the proper care. Even though there are many situations in which you must request additional resources to extricate the patients, you still have several items in your toolbox to extricate the patient.

> **Learning Objectives**
> Upon completing this section, you should be able to
>
> - *understand* how each extrication method is performed,
> - *identify* which extrication device is indicated in a given situation,
> - *infer* the risks of each extrication method,
> - *communicate* when additional resources are required for extrication.

Emergency Extrication

We will begin with the most basic and yet most urgent type of extraction, emergency extraction. Emergency extractions are to be performed in the event where the environment is extremely dangerous for the patient and it can lead to imminent death if left in that environment. An example of this would be a fire or a shooting. Keep in mind that these techniques do not take into account any cervical spine precautions. Additionally, these extraction techniques can be performed without any additional equipment.

© The Author(s), under exclusive license to Springer Nature
Switzerland AG 2021
C. Ventura et al., *The Emergency Medical Responder*,
https://doi.org/10.1007/978-3-030-64396-6_23

One method of emergency extraction is known as the emergency drag. In this technique, your patient will be on the ground. You stand at the patient's head and place each arm under their armpits. You will then wrap your arms tightly around their chest and link your arms. You can then drag the patient out of the environment. One can also perform an emergency drag by grabbing the patient's shirt or jacket at the shoulders and dragging the patient to a safe environment just as you would with the previous emergency drag method.

Building Extraction
Say you are called to respond to a patient at a dorm at your local college. You arrive to find that the patient has a right tibia fracture and cannot ambulate themselves at all. The patient is on the third floor of the dorm building, and no, there is no elevator. How are we going to move the patient to the ambulance? It will be very difficult to carry any type of stretcher with a patient in it up those flights of stars. Thankfully, we have just the tool, the aptly named stair chair. The stair chair is a wheelchair which has handles at the head of the chair as well as the base of the chair to allow EMS providers to move the patient down a flight of stairs while keeping the patient in an upright position. Newer models also have a track system on the bottom; thus, it can be moved down stairs without the EMS provider holding the patient in the air. When using the track system, ensure the track is in contract with multiple stairs. Also, note that the straps should be applied in an X formation across the patient's chest.

When working within a building, you must consider that a common location to find your patient would be in a bed whether it be their own bed at home or in a hospital bed. When a patient is in a bed, it is often best to perform a bed transfer. You may have access to a transfer sheet. A transfer sheet is made of a durable material with handles on each side. In order to use the transfer sheet, you must roll the patient to the side and push the transfer sheet under the patient. You can then roll the patient in the other direction and pull the transfer sheet completely into place. As a team, you and your partners can now more easily move the patient to the stretcher. If a transfer sheet is not available, you may substitute with a standard sheet or blanket.

Vehicle Extraction
When looking at how to extricate a patient from a vehicle as just an emergency medical responder, you can be very limited in what you can do. The primary method of extraction which you can actually do is extraction via the Kendrick Extrication Device which was discussed in a previous chapter. It is important to keep in mind that the process does take a significant amount of time and can only be done in a stable environment.

The main objective when dealing with a vehicle extraction is to immediately call for additional resources and describe the situation as well as any hazards so that the brought equipment can be brought to the scene. As an EMT, attempt to get at least some access to the patient to perform a limited primary assessment. This may involve such things as breaking windows. Also, try not to forget basic things like asking the patient to unlock the door if they can before breaking a window. There will be cases in which you may have to just pull the patient out of the car such as in the event of cardiac arrest, but always remember that your safety is of utmost importance.

Wilderness Extraction
One environment in which you may find yourself in is the not-so-great outdoors. Wilderness response is often regulated to rescue squads and wilderness EMTs, but we will discuss these types of patient extractions in the case you do work in these squads, but remember not to perform any actions you are not trained, certified, and licensed to do.

One environment in which wilderness extractions may be necessary is in a mountainous terrain. In this case, the rescuer may use a smaller EMS pack than your traditional set of gear. These packs often include such things as an AED, oxygen, and a limited trauma bag. The rescuer may grapple and repel to the patient with this gear. Special equipment may also be used to move the patient such as a scoop stretcher or stokes or basket-type stretcher. In especially difficult cases, a sked may also be used for patient extraction until a more definite method can be used.

Another common scenario of wilderness rescue is the aquatic environment. In this case, the rescuer may don either a wetsuit in clean water such as a river or a dry suit, with ankle and neck gasket, in a possibly contaminated water environment such as in the event of an urban flood. In regard to securing the patient for extraction, some options that are available are a floating backboard or water litter.

Chapter 24
Appendix: ALS and BLS Integrated Care

Introduction

As you already know, emergency medical services comprise a collaboration among providers with varied skill sets. In Chap. 1, we discussed the various types of EMS clinicians and their respective scope of practices. Oftentimes, BLS and ALS providers must collaborate to provide exceptional pre-hospital care. This chapter will aid you in becoming a better BLS provider and an overall better EMS clinician, by recognizing the need for an ALS intercept and designing your treatment plan with the help of advanced providers.

> **Learning Objectives**
> Upon completing this section, you should be able to
>
> - *understand* differences in scope of practice,
> - *identify* the need for ALS intercept,
> - *infer* when ALS procedures may be indicated,
> - *communicate* with advanced providers.

The ALS Intercept

It's important to recognize that despite EMRs and EMTs are well-trained medical professionals, there are other treatment and assessment options that are typically available to better care for the patient. Requesting for a consultation from an advanced EMT or paramedic (when the requesting crew is only capable of rendering BLS care) is known as an ALS intercept. Intercepts can typically be requested

© The Author(s), under exclusive license to Springer Nature
Switzerland AG 2021
C. Ventura et al., *The Emergency Medical Responder*,
https://doi.org/10.1007/978-3-030-64396-6_24

directly through dispatch without consulting medical direction. Note that once an ALS assessment has been performed and ALS treatment is rendered, continued care and oversight of the patient must be at the ALS level or higher. At no point should care be downgraded from ALS to BLS unless local protocols, standing orders, or medical direction advises.

Knowing when to call ALS intercept is one of the most important intuitive skills a BLS provider can have and often improves with experience. You have the right as a BLS provider to request an ALS intercept or advice from medical direction at any point of a call regardless of the circumstance. There are no penalties for asking for help. So when should you call for ALS? The answer relies on your ability to understand your scope and the scope of ALS providers. For example, if you were called to the scene of an anaphylactic reaction, you may consider requesting ALS before you even arrive. This is because you already know that if this patient's airway rapidly becomes compromised, they may need advanced airway intervention such as intubation. It is your responsibility as a BLS provider to be able to recognize when BLS assessment and intervention may not be effective or appropriate.

Sometimes, the need for ALS intercept isn't always clear toward the beginning of the call or from the provided dispatch information. For example, you may be called to the scene of a motor vehicle collision with three occupants who have unknown injuries. You might only realize midway through your assessment of the last occupant that ALS is needed, and that is perfectly okay! Remember, ALS intercept is always an option.

So when is it a good time to preemptively request ALS as soon as the tone drops? Typically, this occurs if you anticipate that one or more of the ABCs could be compromised and/or if ALS intervention may be indicated.

For example:

- All airway/breathing emergencies (respiratory distress, asthma attack, COPD, etc.)
- Cardiac arrest
- Cardiac emergencies (angina, symptomatic bradycardia/tachycardia, suspected MI, etc.)
- Diabetic seizures
- High-speed collision injuries

To help aid your understanding of how helpful ALS providers can be, take a look at some of the possible ALS interventions. The list is not an extensive scope of practice overview.

Condition	Possible BLS interventions	Possible ALS interventions
Upper airway compromise	OPA/NPA insertion BVM use	Supraglottic airway Intubation Ventilator
Pediatric asthma attack	Oxygen Assist MDI administration Supportive care	Albuterol sulfate and/or ipratropium bromide Nebulized racemic epinephrine
Pain management	Supportive care Oxygen Acetaminophen (PO) *in some states*	Acetaminophen IV Toradol IV Ketamine IV Morphine IV Fentanyl IV
Cardiac arrhythmias	Supportive care Oxygen 12-lead ECG acquisition *in some states*	4/12-lead ECG monitoring and interpretation Atropine IV (for bradycardias) Adenosine IV (for supraventricular tachycardia) Transcutaneous pacing Synchronized cardioversion

Cardiac arrest	Basic life support (BLS)
	   High-quality CPR
	   Automated external defibrillation
	   BVM use
		Advanced cardiac life support (ACLS)
		   Manual defibrillation
		   Epinephrine IV
		   Vasopressin IV
		   Amiodarone IV
		   Rapid sequence intubation
		   Targeted temperature management

As a BLS provider, you may benefit from researching some of these continuing education topics to assist ALS providers while on scene:

- How to spike a bag
- Basic ECG interpretation
- Sellick's maneuver for endotracheal intubation
- Prehospital Trauma Life Support

Chapter 25
Appendix: Ambulance Operations

Introduction

One of the most recognizable symbols of EMS is the ambulance, and as an EMS provider, you may be working on one or even driving one. You may say "Oh I can drive a car so I can drive an ambulance easily." Hold your horses; there are some major differences when operating an ambulance from its size and weight to its sirens. In this chapter, we will talk about legal considerations, how to actually drive an ambulance, and how to deal with an emergency situation. We will talk about rig checks and how to prepare your routes for responding to a patient. Driving an ambulance is partially about a quick response, but what is most important is safety.

> **Learning Objectives**
> Upon completing this section, you should be able to
>
> - *understand legislature regarding ambulance operations,*
> - *identify each of the three types of ambulances,*
> - *infer what hazards may be present during driving,*
> - *communicate any maintenance or safety concerns of ambulance.*

Legal Considerations

As with most aspects within EMS, the first responder must consider the legal ramifications of their actions and be familiar with all applicable legislature. As an ambulance driver, this is even more important as you are responsible for not only the state's ambulance policies but also the general motor vehicle and traffic laws of your state. Each state has variations in their specific legislature, and thus, we will only be covering general guidelines for ambulance operations.

© The Author(s), under exclusive license to Springer Nature   193
Switzerland AG 2021
C. Ventura et al., *The Emergency Medical Responder*,
https://doi.org/10.1007/978-3-030-64396-6_25

Even though you may not be the primary provider in an EMS call, you are still headed by similar standards of care and must understand key ideas such as consent of care. An example of a situation in which this is relevant is if your patient is alert and oriented with no signs of any altered mental status and your partner wants to transport the patient even though the patient refused care and transport. As the ambulance driver, it is your responsibility to understand and explain to your partner that you cannot transport or care for the patient as this would be battery and kidnapping.

You should also keep in mind the law of due regard which is that all of your actions are ones that would be done by a person of your position with the same level of training. This includes giving adequate alert using sirens, not going extremely excessive speeds, and maintaining an alert state at all times. Even though you are driving an ambulance or other emergency vehicle, you are not above the law and for the most part are to follow general traffic laws. The way the laws regarding ambulances work is in the way of exceptions. In other words, it does not say when you have to follow traffic rules, but rather, it states the specific occasions in which you are exempt from traffic rules. As stated previously, the laws regarding this vary as one state may say that you must use lights and sirens for every patient while another may say that you can only use lights and sirens if the patient becomes critical during transport or if there is a paramedic on board.

Ambulance Maneuvers and Driving

We will get to the main event, actually driving an ambulance, but in order to understand how to drive an ambulance, we must first answer the question "how exactly is an ambulance different from your standard Toyota Prius?" The simple answer is that an ambulance is bigger, much bigger, but we have to look into more specific situations, and we can start off by looking at the three different types of ambulances. The three ambulance designations are based on what vehicles serve as the driver's compartment and the style of patient compartment. In addition to the ambulance types, you can further break down each category into a class 1, which is rear wheel drive, and class 2 which is all wheel drive.

Ambulance designations	
Type I	Truck body with detachable separated patient compartment Modular capabilities
Type II	Van body with integrated patient compartment
Type III	Van driver's compartment with detachable separated patient compartment Modular capabilities

Even with the three types and two classes of ambulances, there are aspects which affect the driving experience and technique which all groups have in common. Keep in mind that ambulances are very long, and this will affect your turning radius. This turning radius is quite large, and thus, it is best to avoid runs when possible, but when you do turn, ensure you are clear from cars on both sides of the vehicle and that you have sufficient clearance from barriers. This brings us to the next important topic which is mirror use. When driving an ambulance, remember that mirrors are your friend. This allows you to see a greater area of your ambulance and is of even great importance as your rear visibility is often occluded by what is happening in regard to patient care. Even though mirrors are very helpful, there will be time where they are not enough such as parking or backing up. In this case, you will ask your partner to get out of the ambulance and guide you. Your partner should always be visible in your mirror. You should also make use of your partner if you are attempting to make a difficult turn as they will often have a better view of incoming traffic on the side furthest from you.

We have talked about how ambulances are large in size, but they are also very heavy because of the vehicle itself as well as the additional equipment. The weight of the ambulance will primarily affect the braking distance as well as momentum. As the weight is increased, there is a significantly increased time for the ambulance to come to a stop. In order to compensate for this, you must have increased awareness. When driving, you should be scanning 12 seconds ahead for possible hazards. Additionally, you should ensure you have the car lengths in all directions especially when going highway speeds. A more accurate way of determining the area you should have cleared in front of you is by time and speed. Below 55mph, you should have 2 seconds of stopping time, while above 55 mph, you should have 4 seconds. Just as the braking of the ambulance is affected so is the acceleration time. The extra weight of the ambulance causes there to be a greater time for acceleration. Your accelerations should also be done gradually. This is especially relevant for merging. It is often not considered, but you should consider the patient's comfort in the back as sudden jolts or movements can sometimes exacerbate the situation. Additionally, your partner may be standing or moving around, and it can be difficult to maintain transport while the ambulance is moving. Also, take into account any hazards which may be present and could affect maneuvering or stopping such as rain, reduced visibility, or significant traffic. In these cases, you should increase the amount of reaction distance around you. Most of all, remember to always drive defensively.

Maintenance and Preparation
A major part of ambulance operations is performed outside of an ambulance call. This is known as the preparatory phase. In this phase, you will be conducting what are commonly known as "rig checks." In the rig check, you will be checking not only that all medical equipment is sufficiently stocked but also that mechanical components are functioning properly. This includes checking the engine, the lights and sirens, the brakes, the fuel level, and that all proper maintenance has been performed. If there is a problem regarding the ambulance, it is your responsibility to report it and take the ambulance out of service. Just like patient care must be recorded, all aspects of a rig check must also be recorded. There are two different types of rig checks. These include a quick check and a full check. A quick check is to be performed after each call and goes over all the most used components of the ambulance as well as any components used in the last call. The full check goes over

all components of the ambience, and these are often performed at the beginning of each shift. You may not necessarily think of this, but if you miss part of the maintenance procedures and this negatively affects patient care, you can be charged with negligence.

The other major part of preparation is determining your routes and navigation. Most agencies will use GPS or navigation apps on a phone, but there will be times when this will fail such as if there is a loss of signal or a dead battery. Thus, it is important to know where the map pack is stored in the ambulance. It is also important that you become familiar with your response area such as major areas or highways. When determining your route, you should consider not only which route is quickest but also which route is safest. When possible, attempt to take a route with minimal turns, stops, and residential streets.

Emergency Operations and Special Considerations
The most exciting part of ambulance operations is emergency operations. Emergency operations are when you are responding to an emergency. It is up to the first responder to determine when it is a true emergency as many ambulance exceptions when it comes to traffic laws are only applicable in an emergency situation. The situation will also determine your use of lights and sirens. There are three standard levels of the use of lights and sirens. These can be seen in the figure below.

Modes of transport	
Code 1	No lights or sirens
	Standard affairs
Code 2	Lights but no sirens
	Urgent response or transport
Code 3	Both lights and sirens
	Critical response or transport

Even though there is an outline when each code level should be used, there are instances in which you may need to use a different code. One example is if the patient has a sound sensitivity you may want to use code 1 even if the patient is in a more critical situation. Additionally if you are called to a domestic abuse call, you may want to go turn your lights and sirens off as you wait for law enforcement.

There are some traffic considerations you must make when making use of the exceptions to traffic laws ambulances have in emergency situations. When preparing to go against traffic, ensure that all cars are stopped forehand and know your intentions. Also, you should take precautions when crossing an insertion with a red light. In some areas, you can request dispatch to change the lights on your route beforehand.

Standard Protocols When Crossing an Intersection
1. Siren wail 300 ft. away from intersection.
2. Siren yelp 150 ft. away from intersection.
3. Brake at crosswalk.
4. Airhorn two times.
5. Ensure intersection is safe and clear.
6. Continue across intersection with yelp siren.
7. Clear each lane as you approach.
8. Be prepared for possible approaching vehicles.

Chapter 26
Appendix: Tactical Operations—Active Shooter

Introduction

Mass casualty shootings have become an unfortunate part of history and affect urban, suburban, and rural areas. This chapter will discuss the role of EMS in the warm zone and how to safely navigate an active shooter situation in collaboration with law enforcement.

Learning Objectives
Upon completing this section, you should be able to

- *understand* your role as an EMS provider in the warm zone,
- *identify* scene safety concerns,
- *infer* best practices under fire,
- *communicate* with other agencies as appropriate.

In addition to usual EMS operations, an active shooter situation brings a whole set of its own challenges. Care under fire and other tactical austere conditions is incredibly overwhelming even for the seasoned EMS clinician. The key to reduced risk operations in the warm zone is open communication and collaboration between law enforcement and EMS.

We define *active shooter* as one or more persons who are actively attempting to murder multiple people in a populated region, historically with a firearm. There is often no rationale behind the choice of victims. Active shooters at times wear *ballistic protective equipment*, which encompass all forms of body armor used in a tactical situation. This equipment is intentionally designed as part of the first

© The Author(s), under exclusive license to Springer Nature Switzerland AG 2021
C. Ventura et al., *The Emergency Medical Responder*,
https://doi.org/10.1007/978-3-030-64396-6_26

responder's wardrobe for personal protective equipment. In a tactical situation, we categorize multiple regions of the surrounding area by threat level.

Regions:

- *Cold zone*: region where no significant threat is anticipated given the known information and where additional resources stage and triage and treatment should ideally occur.
- *Warm zone*: a dynamic region where there is a potential for threat, the only area permitted for EMS personnel
- *Hot zone*: region where there is a high likelihood of direct threat
- *Casualty collection point*: region where initial medical stabilization and triage occur.
- *Incident command post*: where incident command operations occur.
- *Point of wound care*: region where patient care is initiated.

Stage I: Preparation

Most of our time is spent in Stage I preparing for a violent incident. This includes standard rig checks, inventory analysis, and continuing education. It is recommended that all agencies encourage all providers to take a Tactical Emergency Casualty Care Course. The following table includes the recommended inventory for one trauma bag when entering an active shooter situation. There should be at least one trauma bag per two providers.

Quantity	Equipment
1	Tape roll
1	Trauma shears
1	Penlight
1	Permanent marker (black)
2	Needle decompression sets (ALS only)
2	4 in Israeli bandages
2	6 in Israeli bandages
4	Pairs of gloves
4	Occlusive dressings
6	Adult/pediatric tourniquets
6	6 in elastic roll
Multiple	NPAs w/ lubricant
10	4X4 gauze

Stage II: Dispatch

Upon notification of an active shooter event at the 911, public safety answering point (PSAP), law enforcement, Fire/EMS, and ideally a tactical response team such as SWAT should immediately be toned out. Fire/EMS should standby until there is law enforcement guidance. Usually, the first law enforcement personnel that arrive serve as the *contact team*, which are teams of 1–2 officers who directly approach the threat to neutralize the situation. It is generally not appropriate for Fire/EMS to accompany the contact team.

Stage III: Response

Once additional law enforcement units arrive, zones have been established, and an incident commander has been recognized, law enforcement officers can formally team up with Fire/EMS to engage patient care in the warm zone. Each patient care unit should consist of 1–2 EMS providers, with 2–4 law enforcement officers. At all times in the warm zone, the EMS providers should be positioned in between at least two law enforcement officers, ready to neutralize a threat coming from the 12 o'clock or 6 o'clock position. Ideally, it is recommended that there are also officers positioned in the 3 o'clock and 9 o'clock position to protect EMS from the left and right.

Tactical patient care recommendations are contained in the mnemonic THREAT:

- T: Threat suppression
- H: Hemorrhage control
- RE: Rapid extrication to safety
- A: Assessment by Fire/EMS
- T: Transport to definitive medical care

It is also important for Fire/EMS to become familiar with the following terms:

- *Clear*: Law enforcement has cleared the area of any direct threat, and the area has been taken into custody and oversight by police.
- *Secure*: Law enforcement has deemed the area reasonably secure of any threat.
- *Cover*: A lawful command by law enforcement to take cover behind a large object, preferably behind a wall or desk in the event of an impending ballistic attack.
- *Concealment*: A lawful command by law enforcement to hide, to be unseen by the attacker.

Additional Fire/EMS units that arrive on scene should stage and wait for orders from the incident commander. It may be appropriate at times for law enforcement officers to transport critical patients to the hospital in their department squad cars. Refer to your local protocols for more information, as this is relatively a novel practice.

Stage IV: Post-Incident

Post-incident debriefing is critical to safeguarding the health and well-being of all staff involved. Agencies are encouraged to consider implementing Critical Incident Stress Debriefing (CISD), which is a form of psychological therapy where mental health professionals coach personnel with processing their thoughts and feelings in a group setting or one-on-one. This typically occurs within 72 hours of the incident and is an incredibly effective tool for supporting the long-term health of all staff involved. Statistically, it is very likely that lives will have been lost due to the attack. Additionally, active shooter incidents tend to have a wide impact across the nation and foster the attention of multiple communities, interest groups, politicians, and nonprofits. There is no form of preparation or training that can fully prepare personnel for entering and leaving a tragic active shooter incident. Access to healthcare, recognizing early warning signs, and early intervention of mental health professionals are critical to the prevention of these domestic terrorist attacks.

Chapter 27
Appendix: License Reciprocity and License Renewal

Introduction

Throughout life, there are many aspects which are not constant, and one of these is where you happen to live. As an EMT, you will want to be able to work in the place you live, and if you move out of state, you must go through its specific department of health in order to obtain licensure in that state. Even if you do not move states, you must also be aware of the requirements to maintain your license as they also vary by state.

> **Learning Objectives**
> Upon completing this section, you should be able to
>
> - *understand* that not all states have the same reciprocity protocols,
> - *identify* the protocols for reciprocity for your state of interest,
> - *infer* possible difficulties when applying for reciprocity,
> - *communicate* your current credentials to each state.

When you want to move states and keep your EMT license or even just work in a different state, you must apply for an EMT license in that state. Often times if you already have an EMT license in one state, you may be able to receive an EMT license via reciprocity. Reciprocity is the process in which a state will issue a license based on the recognition of the EMT license of another state. This is not standard through all 50 states as some require you to state licensure and/or NREMT certification, take additional state-specific coursework, and have affiliation with an in-state EMS agency. Additionally, there are select few that do not offer reciprocity at all,

© The Author(s), under exclusive license to Springer Nature
Switzerland AG 2021
C. Ventura et al., *The Emergency Medical Responder*,
https://doi.org/10.1007/978-3-030-64396-6_27

and you must apply for initial licensure. Below, we have compiled a general requirement guide for reciprocity in each state. Keep in mind that these are dependent on the state's legislature which is subject to change. Almost all states will require you to pay applicable fees, fill out state-specific forms, have current BLS provider certification, and pass a set of background checks.

General Requirements for Reciprocity in Each State

- Alabama

  - Must have prior NREMT certification.
  - Must take Alabama protocol education which must be performed by an Alabama service or regional EMS office.

- Alaska

  - Must have prior NREMT certification or state licensure.

- Arizona

  - Those with NREMT certification and state licensure will receive a temporary EMT license.
  - Must also complete an EMT refresher course within 6 months to acquire full state licensure.

- Arkansas

  - Must have prior NREMT certification or state licensure.

- California

  - Must have prior NREMT certification and state licensure.

- Colorado

  - Does not offer reciprocity, and one must apply for initial licensure which can be acquired with NREMT certification, BLS certification, and proper background checks.

- Connecticut

  - Must have prior NREMT certification or state licensure.

- Delaware

  - Must have prior NREMT certification and state licensure.
  - Must complete the Delaware state reciprocity course.

- Florida

  - Must have prior NREMT certification.
  - Additional testing may be required per the State of Florida.

- Georgia

  - Must have prior NREMT certification.

- Hawaii

  - The state does not offer reciprocity, and in order to apply for initial reciprocity, one must have NREMT certification as well as complete a state-approved course.

- Idaho

  - Must have prior NREMT certification and state licensure.
  - Must secure affiliation with an Idaho EMS agency.
  - Complete the Idaho landing zone officer course.
  - An additional transition course may be required depending on your initial certification course.

- Illinois

  - Must have prior NREMT certification and state licensure.

- Indiana

  - If you hold NREMT certification, you must also have taken a course equivalent to the Indiana-approved curriculum to obtain reciprocity.
  - If you hold state licensure, you must also pass the Indiana state cognitive and psychomotor exams to obtain reciprocity.

- Iowa

  - Must have prior NREMT certification.

- Kansas

  - Must have taken an EMT course equivalent to the Kansas-approved training program and have passed the NREMT cognitive and psychomotor exams.

- Kentucky

  - Must have prior NREMT certification and state licensure.
  - Must complete additional continuing education credits prior to working.

- Louisiana

  - Must have prior NREMT certification.

- Maine

  - Must have prior state licensure.

- Maryland

  - Must have prior state licensure.
  - Must have approved affiliation with a Maryland EMS agency.

- Massachusetts

  - Must have prior NREMT certification and state licensure.

  – If one only has NREMT certification, they may still apply for initial licensure.

- Michigan

    – Must have prior state licensure.
    – You do not need to have current NREMT certification, but you do have to have both the NREMT cognitive and psychomotor exam at least once.

- Minnesota

    – Must have prior NREMT certification.

- Mississippi

    – Must have prior NREMT certification and state licensure.

- Missouri

    – Must have prior NREMT certification.

- Montana

    – Must have prior NREMT certification and state licensure.

- Nebraska

    – The state does not have reciprocity, but one can apply for initial licensure with NREMT certification as proof of an initial certification program that follows the DOT standard curriculum.

- Nevada

    – Must have prior NREMT certification.
    – If one only has state licensure, the cognitive portion of the NREMT exam must also be taken.
    – One must live currently in Nevada, will live in Nevada within six months, must work for a service in an approved Nevada EMS agency, or must take an initial course in Nevada.

- New Hampshire

    – Must have prior state licensure.
    – Must complete NREMT cognitive exam.
    – Must have taken cognitive and psychomotor exams within the past year.
    – Must have live, work, and have pending job in New Hampshire.
    – Initial certification course must meet New Hampshire standard curriculum.

- New Jersey

    – Must have prior NREMT certification or state licensure.
    – Must complete all New Jersey EMT refresher course.

- New Mexico

  - Must have prior NREMT certification and state licensure for the state to issue a temporary license.
  - A New Mexico EMS transition course and written examination must be completed to obtain a full state license.

- New York

  - Must have prior NREMT certification or state licensure.
  - NREMT or state-approved cognitive and psychomotor testing within the last 18 months.

- North Carolina

  - Must have prior NREMT certification.
  - Must also reside in the state or have a letter of a conditional job offer from an EMS agency within the state.

- North Dakota

  - Must have prior NREMT certification.

- Ohio

  - Must have prior NREMT certification.
  - Additional coursework may be required depending on your initial certification course.

- Oklahoma

  - Must have prior NREMT certification.

- Oregon

  - Must have prior NREMT certification and state licensure.
  - Must also provide a high school diploma or equivalent.

- Pennsylvania

  - Must have prior NREMT certification.

- Rhode Island.

  - Must either have current NREMT certification, or you may use a current state licensure to challenge and sit for the Rhode Island EMT exam to gain reciprocity.

- South Carolina

  - Must have prior NREMT certification or state licensure.

- South Dakota

  - Must either have current NREMT certification or have been NREMT certified in the past.
  - If your NREMT certification has lapsed, you must provide proof of current state licensure.

- Tennessee

  - Must have prior NREMT certification and state licensure.

- Texas

  - Must have prior state licensure.
  - Must either have NREMT certification or take the NREMT assessment exam.

- Utah

  - Must have prior NREMT certification and state licensure.
  - Must complete state-approved refresher course.

- Vermont

  - Must have prior NREMT certification.
  - The state also requires that you be sponsored by an EMS agency or medical facility where you plan to work which requires that level of licensure.

- Virginia

  - Must have prior NREMT certification or state licensure.
  - Must also complete Virginia continuing education and take cognitive exam within 1 year.

- Washington

  - Initial licensure application is used for reciprocity.
  - Must have prior NREMT certification and state licensure.
  - Proof of completion of an approved training program.

- West Virginia

  - Must have prior NREMT certification or state licensure with 1 year remaining before expiration.
  - Must also either provide proof in additional competencies or undergo an education program of competencies such as MCI, hazmat training, and West Virginia EMS protocols.

- Wisconsin

  - Must have prior NREMT certification and state licensure.
  - Must also provide proof of completion of the Wisconsin MCI course.

- Wyoming

  - The state does not offer reciprocity, but one can use an NREMT certification to receive approval to sit for the state EMT exam and obtain state licensure.

As the influence and usage of the National Registry of Emergency Medical Technicians continue to grow, it may also be important to consider how one can apply for NREMT certification with a current state licensure. Though the NREMT is used widely throughout the United States, remember that it is a private organization and thus does not have the authority to allow one to work in a given state. One must also obtain licensure in the state to practice.

Reciprocity for NREMT Certification
1. Successful completion of a state-approved EMT course within 2 years or, if it has been more than 2 years from the date of completion for the initial state-approved EMT course, one may complete either a state-approved EMT refresher course or 24 hours of equivalent continuing education credits within the past 2 years.
2. Possess BLS for the healthcare provider.
3. Pass both the NREMT cognitive exam and state psychomotor exam.
4. Pay applicable application fees.

Once you obtain your initial state licensure, you do not set for life, but rather, you must continue learning. Every state will vary in what they require to maintain your licensure and will have their own set of continuing education. Some states may just require you to maintain your NREMT certification. NREMT recertification can be obtained in two ways, the first of which is via examination. In this case, you have one attempt to pass the NREMT exam. The other method is to recertify by continuing education. In this case, you must complete 40 hours of continuing education credits, and these must be completed in a specific distribution in three components. Seven hours in each category can be distributive which is where the instructor and student do not meet face-to-face such as in online courses. The exception is the individual component which can be completely distributive.

NREMT Recertification by Continuing Education
National component (20 hrs)

- Airway/respiration/ventilation: 1.5 hours
- Cardiovascular: 6 hours
- Trauma: 1.5 hours
- Medical: 6 hours
- Operations: 5 hours

State component (10 hrs)

- These courses are dependent on what is specified by each individual state. If it is not specified, you may use any state- or CAPCE-approved EMS continuing education course to fulfill this requirement.

Individual component (10 hrs)

- You may use any state- or CAPCE-approved EMS continuing education course to fulfill this requirement.

Chapter 28
Appendix: Neurophysiology for the EMS Provider

Introduction

In Chap. 4, we discussed various clinical presentations of neurological emergencies you may encounter out in the field. As we are already familiar with, the central nervous system is a complex network of neuronal pathways that transfer critical information from multiple relay points. In this appendix chapter, you will begin to better appreciate the complex inner workings of the central and peripheral nervous system as we provide an academic-based introductory overview to the fundamentals of neurophysiology at the molecular level. A general background in biology or chemistry is recommended for optimal engagement but certainly not required. This is a continuing education topic and is not included in the NHTSA curriculum for the EMT-B.

Learning Objectives
Upon completing this section, you should be able to

- *understand* the role of neuronal connections,
- *identify* various neural networks,
- *infer* how neurophysiology can affect a patient's overall condition,
- *communicate* the function of common neurotransmitters.

Introduction
Contemporary neuroscience shepherds the intersection between biopsychology and data science. To best understand how neuronal connections correspond with a meaningful human experience, we must initially reduce these complex networks into a more simplified fundamental concept—connections. The central nervous system is all about relationships and faithful communication between cells. Propagation

C. Ventura et al., *The Emergency Medical Responder*, https://doi.org/10.1007/978-3-030-64396-6_28

patterns of action potentials, membrane potentials, and interneurons and the utilization of third party catalysts and transport proteins all dictate how loyal these neuronal correspondences are received. This appendix chapter will provide an intuitive-driven overview on the neurochemical and biological constituents of the brain's meticulous "telephone game-like" system and will discuss implications for neuropharmacological interventions, pathology, and plasticity.

More on Connections
We will refer to transmitting and receiving neurons as cells. We say that a cell that transmits a neurochemical in the human brain is "presynaptic" and its receiving counterpart is "postsynaptic." Presynaptic and postsynaptic cells can be neurons, tissue cells, muscle cells, or any cell that responds to the neuro-stimulus in question. When a presynaptic cell is a neuron, its transmitting action potential is either excitatory or inhibitory where its resulting effects influence an individual cell or a larger system. It is critical that we preface by explicitly imposing a gross oversimplification of nerve networks into a mere reduction of elementary connections and relationships to build an intuition that supports the convention of biology and standard data processing—and this makes sense. Much like computer circuits, the brain uses the facilitation of specialized pathways to influence the resulting effects of a transmission. Neuronal connections can converge and diverge into singular or multiple pathways as a method of modulating the "strength" of a signal. Additionally, inhibitory and excitatory feedback loops are employed, as well as methods of horizontal and lateral inhibition that support the intentions of the pathway.

Diffuse Modulatory Systems
Aside from pathways architectured for organized synaptic direction and intention, diffuse modulatory systems allow for a signal to be diffusely disseminated across a system. When we think about oxytocin and dopamine flooding the brain postorgasm or the broad effects of cocaine on the central nervous system, we are acknowledging the workings of diffuse modulatory systems. These systems are, in essence, groups of neurons on the order of thousands that synapse onto axons of other neurons. Each neuron of a singular group can influence over 100,000 postsynaptic cells that project almost everywhere. This means that neurochemicals that travel through these systems have more varied and generalized effects than traditional ones. Popular culture has often introduced more well-known neurochemicals such as dopamine and serotonin because of their recognizable effects attributed to dopaminergic and serotonergic diffuse modulatory systems. Similarly, there are also noradrenergic and cholinergic systems that correspond with noradrenaline and acetylcholine, respectively.

Defining Neurochemicals
We say that chemical compounds whose molecular structure—particularly its functional groups—serves as a signaling molecule or stimulus to a neuronal receptor have the potential to be a neurochemical, such that further and more definitive criteria exist to concisely identify legitimate neurochemicals (which for our purpose we can refer to interchangeably as neurotransmitters). Neurochemicals exist when they (i) are in

the presynaptic terminus; (ii) are released when the presynaptic cell is electrically stimulated; (iii) are bound to a postsynaptic cell, where it elicits an excitatory post-synaptic potential (EPSP) or inhibitory postsynaptic potential (IPSP); and (iv) have a receptor in the postsynaptic membrane and (v) there exists a mechanism to remove the chemical from activation in the synaptic cleft such as reuptake or enzymatic degradation. Intermolecular forces and interactions with receptor and neurochemical functional groups such as hydroxyl, amino, and carbonyl groups are key players in specific functions of neurochemicals. Dipole-dipole interactions dictated by strong electronegativity differences have the potential to change receptor protein structures, which also contribute to the response cascade once a receptor is activated or initiated.

Neuropeptides

While neurochemicals are traditionally synthesized in the axon terminal of presynaptic neurons, neuropeptides are created in the soma of the neuron and stored in vesicles within the axon terminal. Synthesis is remarkably similar to general protein synthesis involving DNA transcription and translation. Neuropeptides, generally 3–36 amino acids in length, serve as co-transmitters that are released from a presynaptic cell when strong repeated signals of action potentials are propagated. One neuropeptide is typically released with every one conventional neurotransmitters to modify the action of the neurotransmitter. Unlike typical neurochemicals, neuropeptides can change metabolic machinery and alter gene expression. Effects produced by neuropeptides are slow-acting and have a prolonged response.

Biosynthesis of Neurochemicals in the Presynaptic Cell

The anabolism of neurochemicals is a stepwise biochemical process that relies on highly specific enzymes to move the reaction forward. In the acetylcholine story, ion-gated channels allow choline to enter the presynaptic axon terminal to be met with acetyl coenzyme A to produce acetylcholine stored in vesicles, facilitated by the catalyst acetylcholine transferase. Voltage-gated ion channels open and allow for an influx of calcium ions in this subsequent step, which in turn allow for the fusion of the vesicle to the axon terminal and the release of acetylcholine into the synaptic cleft via exocytosis. Neurons whose architecture revolve around the biosynthesis of specific neurochemicals have their respective specialized catalysts and precursor compounds at all times. In fact, precursor compounds are often recycled by forward and reverse reactions that occur secondary to a reuptake mechanism. For example, the enzyme acetylcholinesterase catabolizes acetylcholine made in excess into choline and acetate to be reused in continued biosynthesis.

The biosynthesis of catecholamines is particularly unique in that there are multiple chemical products that serve as neurochemicals, namely, dopamine (DA), norepinephrine (NE), and epinephrine (EPI). Continued or inhibited production of the pathway will trivially result in varied outcomes. This becomes of increasing interest in terms of neuropharmacology. Suppose a drug entitled "CHRISTIANelenol," generic for "Christianagra," inhibits the enzyme dopamine 3-hydroxylase which in the normal mammalian brain converts DA to NE. Not only would the production of NE be inhibited, but also would EPI. While targeted inhibition via pharmacological intervention is not a novel concept, it emphasizes a fundamental notion that neuronal connections and pathways can be manipulated. Internal biological mechanisms can also participate in the manipulation of a pathway. Kinase enzymes, for example, phosphorylate transmembrane receptors by transferring highly negative phosphate groups to them, which in turn can cause conformational structural changes in proteins, whereby making kinases an effective biological switch to activate or deactivate a pathway.

Receptor Types in the Postsynaptic Cell

Most neurochemicals subscribe to the use of one or both of two types of ligand-gated transmembrane receptors in the postsynaptic cell: ionotropic and metabotropic receptors. Ionotropic receptors work by binding to a signal molecule which opens an ion channel. When ions diffuse across an electrochemical gradient, the cell will either hyperpolarize or depolarize which corresponds to the likelihood of action potential propagation.

Metabotropic receptors likewise bind to a signal molecule; however, this gives rise to a shape change in G-coupled proteins that can influence enzymatic activity, gene transcription, and the opening of other ion channels through secondary messaging. We attribute complex signaling cascades most often to metabotropic receptors.

Selective Serotonin Reuptake Inhibition

An estimated 17.3 million adults in the United States have experienced major depression with an annual increasing trend (NIH 2017). Of this population, over 44% use medication as a method of treatment. According to a 2017 meta-analysis review, it has become increasingly evident that selective serotonin reuptake inhibitors (SSRIs) are significantly more beneficial in treating depression combined with regular therapy when compared to placebo. While the exact mechanism of action for SSRIs is not entirely understood, it is hypothesized that the drug inhibits the reuptake mechanism of serotonin in the presynaptic cell, thus increasing the quantity and duration of serotonin in the synaptic cleft which through some unknown mechanism increases mood and inevitably decreases the severity and frequency of depression-type symptoms. Because serotonin travels via the serotonergic diffuse modulatory pathway, increasing the quantity and duration of serotonin in the synapse increases the effects of serotonin throughout the entire central nervous system.

This system also accounts for most known adverse effects including insomnia, loss of appetite, and sexual dysfunction. Sexual desire is often a significant complaint among SSRI users because the overwhelming occupancy of serotonin in multiple synapses inhibits the available surface area for libido-promoting hormones to reach these synapses. This simultaneously decreases the likelihood of sexual arousal and raises the threshold of reaching orgasm.

The Need for Continued Research
Much like social networking, the brain heavily relies on precise interactions that can have varied amplitudes of impact across a system. And similarly, this system is susceptible to third-party manipulation, malfunction, and regular system upgrades. The construction of pathways in the CNS and its specific compound to receptor interactions heavily relies on biochemistry. Van der Waals interactions between functional groups of neurochemicals and transmembrane protein receptors in particular have postsynaptic ramifications and are highly influential in activating protein shape changes. It is glaringly undeniable that continued research is warranted to further investigate mechanisms of action of psychoactive pharmacology, affinity and conditions of critical catalysts, and the role epigenetics has on influencing neuronal systems as a whole.

It is important for prehospital providers to have some degree of familiarity with neurophysiology, to best appreciate how the presence of pathology in neuronal connections translate to recognizable symptomatology.

Chapter 29
Appendix: Accessibility in EMS Education

Introduction

This chapter identifies key issues regarding accessibility in emergency care classrooms that provide cardiopulmonary resuscitation (CPR) and first aid training and suggests potential solutions for promoting a positive, safe, and inclusive learning environment. These solutions may encourage bystander intervention and in turn improve outcomes of patients who rely on competent rescuers.

> **Learning Objectives**
> Upon completing this section, you should be able to
>
> - *understand* best practices for maintaining an accessible classroom,
> - *identify* the need for continued learning on accessibility and inclusion,
> - *infer* appropriate alternatives to traditional psychomotor testing.

Hundreds of thousands of individuals across the globe are mandated to keep up their CPR or first aid certification up to date as an occupational requirement. This is typically satisfied by successfully completing the appropriate program that complies with the recent International Liaison Committee on Resuscitation (ILCOR) science, such as a program offered through the American Heart Association, the American Safety and Health Institute, or the Heart and Stroke Foundation of Canada.

CPR and first aid instructors are tasked with the honor and responsibility of educating community members and healthcare providers with lifesaving skills and science that affect survival outcomes of sudden cardiac arrest victims. This goes without saying that the student population is as diverse as any, from daycare

© The Author(s), under exclusive license to Springer Nature
Switzerland AG 2021
C. Ventura et al., *The Emergency Medical Responder*,
https://doi.org/10.1007/978-3-030-64396-6_29

teachers to critical care nurses. Concurrently, according to the Centers for Disease Control, one in four adults in the United States have some type of disability. This comes as no shock to the seasoned instructor, balancing the need to check for high-quality chest compressions while complying with accessibility education laws and regulations.

This is an inevitable challenge that many instructors come across, compensating the key question "If a student is unable to perform these skills in the classroom, are they able to perform them in a true emergency? If not, am I obligated to issue certification?" Usually in an attempt to answer this question, training providers advise legal counsel or encourage instructors to use their best judgment. However, advising instructors to utilize best judgment results in incontinuity of course conduction and ultimately a variance course quality. The following suggests potential solutions to accessibility issues in the emergency care classroom.

General Accessibility Considerations

An ideal emergency care classroom environment promotes positive, safe, and inclusive learning to improve outcomes of patients who are the victims of life-threatening illnesses. Facilities should be well lit, have restroom access, and appeal to audio, visual, and hands-on learners. If the facility is unable to provide food or beverage, instructors should consider allowing students to bring their own light snacks for students who have strict dietary schedules or are diabetic. Training facilities may consider including a statement advising students to notify the facility in advance of a disability so the appropriate accommodations can be planned for. It is encouraged for instructors to uphold, promote, and advertise his or her commitment to accessible and inclusive learning.

Temporary Injuries

Should a student present with a temporary injury that disables them from adequately participating in skill sessions, such as an upper extremity injury that disallows for adequate chest compression depth, we suggest allowing the student to complete the entire duration of the course while temporarily withholding certification. If the course is required for employment, instructors might consider writing a letter to the employer detailing their participation in the didactic portion or the successful completion of the required exam and invite the student to return within 30 days to complete the skills portion.

Knee and Back Issues

Instructors should attempt to accommodate students with knee or back issues by providing kneeling mats for CPR skills practice or allowing the student to conduct the skill on a stretcher or table. Real-life approaches such as the use of CPR stools or lowering a stretcher device to an accessible height level may be beneficial to the student's experience.

Deaf and Hard of Hearing
For students with auditory disabilities, consideration of using a qualified interpreter may be beneficial. If an instructor is made aware in advance of students with auditory disabilities, the instructor may consider investing in an automated external defibrillator trainer that has additional visual prompts.

Learning Disabilities
If a written exam is required, students with test anxiety or other testing-related disability might benefit from extended time by multiplying the allotted test-taking time by 1.5 if possible. Taking the exam in isolation from other students may improve the student's confidence, decrease associated anxiety, and decrease the opportunity for distractions. For dyslexic students, instructors may consider contacting their training provider if a dyslexia-assisting software can be used during an exam. If not, instructors should consider reading aloud the questions and answer choices.

In any event, during psychomotor testing, students should be given equal responsibility to timely response, activation of the emergency response system, and high-quality performance of the necessary skills. Instructors should always follow the guidelines of the training provider they are credentialed under first and foremost. If students are unable to satisfy skill requirements after appropriate accessibility accommodations are exhausted, certification which testifies student proficiency in the course curriculum standards may not be appropriately warranted.

Educators who commit to accessibility and inclusion in the classroom assure a community of competent rescuers, may increase the likelihood of bystander intervention, and may overall improve the survival and quality-of-life outcomes of patients who rely on the delivery of the science.

Chapter 30
Appendix Practice Exam

Before You Begin
- Write your answers on a sheet of paper.
- Time yourself; aim to finish before 1.5 hours.
- Use the score analysis tool at the end of the exam to see how you did!
- These questions are primarily for your own use as most content will not be tested on during your national registry or state exam.

1. Which of these patients should you triage as green?

    (a) 50-year-old male who is on the floor with a broken ankle and cannot walk
    (b) 12-year-old boy who is unresponsive and without a pulse or breathing
    (c) 60-year-old woman who walks up to you and says she can't feel her arm
    (d) 40-year-old man on the floor unconscious with no other signs of trauma

2. Which of these is an ALS drug which may be administered when treating a patient with supraventricular tachycardia?

    (a) Adenosine
    (b) Oral glucose
    (c) Toradol
    (d) Naproxen

3. The hot zone is best defined as the:

    (a) region where no significant threat is anticipated given the known information
    (b) region right outside a burning building

C. Ventura et al., *The Emergency Medical Responder*, https://doi.org/10.1007/978-3-030-64396-6_30

      (c) region where there is a high likelihood of direct threat

      (d) region where there is a potential for threat, the only area permitted for EMS personnel

4. Which patient extraction devices would be recommended in an aquatic rescue?

      (a) Kendrick Extrication Device

      (b) Stair chair

      (c) Stokes stretcher

      (d) Water litter

5. You arrive at the scene of a major traffic accident involving a bus and three other cars. There are a large number of injured patients. What is the first task to be performed?

      (a) Establish an incident commander.

      (b) Count how many patients you have at the scene.

      (c) Call all the patients and ask them to walk to you to see if they can ambulate.

      (d) Begin treating the patient you think is most critical.

6. You arrive on scene to a 50-year-old male patient who has a severe head pain. He describes it as his head is exploding. The patient also complains of sensitivity to loud noises. The patient appears to be becoming more critical. What would be the best code to transport the patient at?

      (a) Code 1

      (b) Code 2

      (c) Code 3

      (d) Code 4

7. Which of the following is **not** a possible difficulty to consider when driving an ambulance?

      (a) Decreased ability to accelerate.

      (b) Increased braking time.

      (c) Low rear visibility.

      (d) All of the above should be considered.

8. Which of the following is part of the THREAT mnemonic for tactical operations:

      (a) Attack the shooter.

      (b) Rapid extrication to safety.

      (c) Remain calm.

      (d) Treat your patient.

9. What organization manages ICS classes and certifications?

      (a) AHA

      (b) NREMT

      (c) FEMA

      (d) State EMS office

10. Your ambulance has a truck-style driver's compartment with a removable and modular patient compartment. What class is this ambulance?

(a) Class 1
(b) Class 2
(c) Class 3
(d) Class 4

11. What is the last stage of an active shooter EMS response?

(a) Clearing
(b) Dispatch
(c) Post-incident
(d) Response

12. How many areas of continuing education are required by the NREMT to renew your certification?

(a) 3
(b) 1
(c) 5
(d) 2

13. The treatment for organophosphate poisoning is:

(a) Atropine
(b) Epinephrine
(c) Ibuprofen
(d) Naloxone

14. Which of the following is an ALS airway management technique?

(a) Endotracheal intubation
(b) Oropharyngeal airway
(c) Nasopharyngeal airway
(d) Head-tilt/chin-lift maneuver

15. You are teaching a CPR class to a group of teachers. One has a broken arm and says she needs certification this week for work. What would **not** be an acceptable way to resolve the situation?

(a) Offer to write a letter to her employer.
(b) Allow her to return in 30 days to complete the skills portion.
(c) Issue her the certification anyway.
(d) Temporarily withhold the certification until their skills can be verified.

16. Which of the following is not a symptom or sign of organophosphate poisoning?

(a) Urination
(b) Lacrimation
(c) Salivation
(d) Constipation

17. How many seconds ahead should you scan when driving an ambulance on the highway?

(a) 60 seconds
(b) 2 seconds
(c) 4 seconds
(d) 15 seconds

18. Which of the following does not function as a neurotransmitter?

(a) Dopamine
(b) Epinephrine
(c) Norepinephrine
(d) Tyrosine

19. You find that one of the accelerometer gauges is not functioning when you perform the rig check at the beginning of your shift. What would the proper thing to do be?

(a) Report your findings and take the ambulance out of service.
(b) Continue with your shift and estimate your speed.
(c) Attempt to fix the gauge yourself.
(d) None of the above.

20. Why is it important to triage patients during an MCI event?

(a) To ensure there are no additional threats.
(b) To determine how to allocate limited resources to a large group of patients.
(c) The states like to not waste money unnecessarily.
(d) You need to document how many patients are at the scene.

21. Which of these is not true of the NREMT?

(a) They aid in the testing process of EMS education.
(b) You only have one attempt to renew your certification via the cognitive test.
(c) NREMT certification is required by several states in order to gain reciprocity issued.
(d) The NREMT can give you permission to practice in a state without approval from the state EMS office.

22. A group of patients who all rode a specific train report severe nausea and pain several weeks later. Which is the most likely used weapon of mass destruction type.

(a) Explosive
(b) Biological
(c) Chemical
(d) Radiological

23. A cell that transmits a neurochemical in the human brain is described as:

   (a) Presynaptic
   (b) Postsynaptic
   (c) Synaptic
   (d) Anti-synaptic

24. You respond and are involved in an active shooter situation, and you begin to come under fire. You can see the shooter approaching. You react by hiding in a bush. You are said to be taking:

   (a) Clearance
   (b) Cover
   (c) Concealment
   (d) Protection

25. Which of the following should be looked at during a full rig check?

   (a) The pressure of the main ambulance oxygen tank
   (b) The functioning of all sirens and lights
   (c) The ambulance tire pressures
   (d) All of the above

Practice Test Answer Key

   1. c
   2. a
   3. c
   4. d
   5. a
   6. b
   7. d
   8. b
   9. c
  10. a
  11. c
  12. a
  13. a
  14. a
  15. c
  16. d
  17. c

18. d
19. a
20. b
21. d
22. d
23. a
24. c
25. d

No. of questions correct	Score + recommendation
23–25	Great job! You really know your stuff!
20–23	Pretty good! You seem to have studied a lot, but you may have one or two
17–20	areas where you may not be completely comfortable in.
0–17	Pass: you did ok, but it is recommended that you continue to review the
	information to gain a full mastery as you have areas of weakness.
	Fail: you have not shown sufficient competency in these areas of study. It is
	recommended that you really hit the books to learn the information.

Chapter Practice Questions Answer Key

Chapter 1

1. C
2. A
3. A

Chapter 2

1. C
2. B
3. B
4. A

Chapter 3

1. C
2. C
3. D
4. B

Chapter 4

1. B
2. A
3. C

Chapter 5

1. A
2. B
3. D
4. A

Chapter 6

1. A
2. A
3. A
4. A

Chapter 7

1. B
2. B
3. C
4. C

Chapter 8

1. A
2. C
3. B
4. D

Chapter 11

1. B
2. D
3. D

Chapter 13

1. B
2. C
3. B

Chapter 14

1. C
2. B
3. C

Chapter 15

1. D
2. C
3. D

Chapter 16

1. C
2. B
3. D

References

1. National Standard Curriculum for EMT-Basic training by the National Highway Traffic Safety Administration (NHTSA).
2. Stoy WA, et al. Mosby's EMT-basic textbook: Mosby Lifeline; 2011.
3. Barnes L, et al. Emergency care and transportation of the sick and injured: Jones & Bartlett Learning; 2015.
4. National Registry of Emergency Medical Technicians "Patient Assessment / Management – Trauma", "Patient Assessment / Management – Medical".
5. American Heart Association, International Liaison Committee on Resuscitation (ILCOR) "Emergency Cardiovascular Care CPR & First-Aid Guidelines".
6. National Association of Emergency Medical Technicians, American College of Surgeons "Prehospital Trauma Life Support Guidelines".
7. National Registry of Emergency Medical Technicians., NREMT.org
8. Ventura C, et al. An overview of emergency medical services pandemic response in the United States and its implications during the era of COVID-19. SSRN Electron J. 2020 https://doi.org/10.2139/ssrn.3631136.
9. Ventura C, et al. Emergency medical services resource capacity and competency amid COVID-19 in the United States: preliminary findings from a National Survey. Heliyon. 2020;6(5) https://doi.org/10.1016/j.heliyon.2020.e03900.
10. Ventura C. Are EMS agencies contributing to the spread of COVID-19 in the U.S.? The fault lays on our policies. The problem, the solution and how we go from here. J Emerg Med Serv. 2020;
11. U.S Fire Administration: Fire/Emergency Medical Services Department Operational Considerations and Guide for Active Shooter and Mass Casualty Incidents (September, 2013).
12. National Association of Emergency Medical Technician "Tactical Emergency Casualty Care Guidelines".
13. Hazinski MF. Basic life support (BLS) provider manual: American Heart Association; 2016.
14. Advanced Cardiovascular Life Support (ACLS): Provider manual. American Heart Association, 2016.
15. "Best Practices for Protecting EMS Responders during Treatment and Transport of Victims of Hazardous Substance Releases." Occupational Safety and Health Administration, U.S. Department of Labor, 2009.
16. Fire / Emergency Medical Services Department Operational Considerations and Guide for Active Shooter and Mass Casualty Incidents. Federal Emergency Management Agency, 2013.

Index

© The Author(s), under exclusive license to Springer Nature
Switzerland AG 2021
C. Ventura et al., *The Emergency Medical Responder*,
https://doi.org/10.1007/978-3-030-64396-6

GPSR Compliance

The European Union's (EU) General Product Safety Regulation (GPSR) is a set of rules that requires consumer products to be safe and our obligations to ensure this.

If you have any concerns about our products, you can contact us on ProductSafety@springernature.com

In case Publisher is established outside the EU, the EU authorized representative is:

Springer Nature Customer Service Center GmbH
Europaplatz 3
69115 Heidelberg, Germany

Batch number: 10091867

Printed by Printforce, the Netherlands